BLAKE POWELL'S
WELL-FIT BOOK

Dedication

To my wife, Mary, and my children, Anathea and Patrick, for the love, support, and encouragement they gave me while I worked on this book.

Blake Powell's
WELL-FIT BOOK

Blake Powell, M.D.
Carlisle Hospital
Carlisle, Pennsylvania

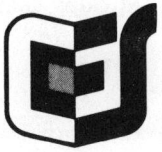

GEORGE F. STICKLEY COMPANY
210 W. Washington Square, Philadelphia, PA

Acknowledgment

I thank Donna Rentzel of the Department of Emergency Medicine, Milton S. Hershey Medical Center, Hershey, Pennsylvania, for her skilled typing and helpful support, and the personnel of Fitness America, York, Pennsylvania, for being the models in the photographs.

RA
776.5
.P6

Copyright © by the George F. Stickley Company
ISBN-89313-037-0
Library of Congress Card # 83-061167

All Rights Reserved. No part of this book may be reproduced in any form without permission from the publisher.

Printed and Manufactured in the United States and published by the George F. Stickley Company, 210 West Washington Square, Philadelphia, Pa. 19106.

Contents

Prologue ix
    The First Step • Basis of Book • The Well-Fit Way

1   Those Mysterious Myths 1
No Control Over Health • Can't Understand Your Body • Pill for Every Ill • Anything Can be Fixed (and Instantly) • Four Free's • Perfection • Why We Believe Those Things • Well-Fit Tips

2   Killing Softly 5
National Problem • Money • Your Problem • Well-Fit Tips

3   Wellness 9
Looking Ahead • Self-Respect • Benefits • Well-Fit Tips

4   Your Condition 12
Health Hazard Appraisal • Your Present Body • Fat • Conditioning • Well-Fit Tips

5 Look Before Leaping 18
Heart Problem Signs • Check-up • Well-Fit Tips

6 Smoking 21
What is It • How it Hurts You • Stopping • Well-Fit Tips

7 Alcohol And Other Drugs 25
What is It • How it Hurts You • Moderation • Well-Fit Tips

8 Stress 28
What is It • What It Does to You • Problems • Well-Fit Tips

9 Well-Fit Stress 32
Stress Management • Relaxation Response • Benefits • Well-Fit Tips

10 Bad Food 36
American Diet • Refined Foods • Fat • Sugar • Fiber • Health Problems • Well-Fit Tips

11 Well-Fit Food 41
Good Nutrition • Unrefined Foods • Fiber • Protein/Fat/ Carbohydrate Balance • Vitamins/Minerals • Fluids • Well-Fit Tips

12 Fat 46
Your Body Fat • Lean/Fat Mass • Problems • Well-Fit Tips

13 Well-Fit Weight 49
Ideal Weight • Ideal Fat Content • Well-Fit Tips

CONTENTS

14   **Exercise** 52
What is It • What It Does • How It Helps • Well-Fit Tips

15   **Well-Fit Exercise** 55
Max. Heart Rate • LSD • Target Zone • Well-Fit Tips

16   **Well-Fit Program** 58
Twelve Weeks to Change • Positive Feedback • Finding Time • Well-Fit Triad • Well-Fit Tips

17   **Well-Fit Way—Reasonable Rest** 61
Using Stress Management • Time-Outs • Well-Fit Tips

18   **Well-Fit Way—Regulated Weight** 63
Caloric Need • Losing Weight • Maintaining Weight • Exchange Lists • Behavior Modification • Well-Fit Tips

19   **Well-Fit Way—Rational Exercise** 69
Aerobics • Flexibility • Strength • Things to Do • Following Your Progress • Cycling Training • Well-Fit Tips

20   **Your Neighborhood Resources** 85
Health Spas • Weight Loss Centers • Clubs • Family • Well-Fit Tips

21   **Injury** 88
Over-use • Strains and Sprains • Fractures • Fatigue and Over-Training • Self-Help • Well-Fit Tips

22   **Feminine Fitness** 92
Concerns • Pregnancy • Menstruation • Bras • Well-Fit Tips

23   **Body Parts**   94
           Teeth • Back • Well-Fit Tips

24   **Fads**   97
           Life Quality • Life Expectancy • Chance • Well-Fit Tips

25   **Your Well-Fit Lifetime**   103

Epilogue   105
       Thousand Mile Journey

Index   107

Prologue

THE FIRST STEP

This is a guide book, a do-it-yourself book, the book that will show you how to:

increase your life expectancy • have more control over your health • learn how to lose weight and fat and *keep it off* • exercise correctly using short, fun, productive work-outs • handle stress • know what foods to eat • know what to do for your low back pain • do all of this and fit it all into your daily routine.

Using only yourself, a tape measure, a scale, a watch, a pocket calculator, and a few other things, you'll learn how to design and use your own personal program for better health. During the first 12 weeks of your program, you'll lose 10 to 20 pounds, gain fitness, reduce stress, and learn how to eat. That's right, learn *how to eat*.

Everything in these pages is based on scientific fact. No fads, no craziness. This is the product of almost 10 years of study, work, and experiment. I use these methods myself, and I have helped others use them. As a matter of fact, I couldn't count the number of classes, talks, and presentations I have given during the past several years telling people about these methods. Those people are using these techniques because they work.

The basis of this book is that you and everyone else can have a positive influence on your health and life. You already know too well that you can have a negative influence on your health. I see the results every day.

As a specialist in Emergency Medicine, I see the results of self-neglect and self-abuse constantly, and I'm tired of it. There is another way. To get there you have to look ahead with self-respect. You have to *use* fitness for wellness. This book is the Well-Fit Way to better health. I became so upset with the things I was seeing (and still see) in the Emergency Room that I looked around for some other way and found it in my Exercise Physiology and competitive athletic background— *fitness helps to prevent problems.* Fitness helps you to achieve wellness, a state of health much higher than just "not ill." Wellness helps to prevent disease, reduce the effects of an illness if you get one, and give you your optimal life expectancy.

Wellness helps to improve the quality of your life.

So, read on. Learn about yourself. Learn how to be well; how to be fit. Learn how only 20 minutes invested in yourself each day can change your life. Learn how you can watch a movie, or a football game, or even "General Hospital" while you improve your body at the same time.

There is an old Chinese saying—"The beginning of a thousand mile journey is the first step." Remember that proverb. This book is your first step to a life of fitness and wellness. Welcome to the Well-Fit Way. Enjoy it.

1

Those Mysterious Myths

There are a number of mysterious myths believed by many people in this country, myths that create problems. Because of those crazy beliefs, people don't take care of themselves. Let's look at some of them.

Many people, perhaps even you, believe that they don't have any control over their health. All of you couldn't be more wrong! Everyone has a profound influence over his or her body and health. Think about it. You are the only one who can feel your own pain. You are the only one who can fully understand yourself. The rest of us look in from the outside. If you learn to listen more to your own body, you can have more of an influence over it, including helping it to be healthy. Always remember this *myth*, and don't believe it.

The next detrimental belief is that we can't possibly understand ourselves, our bodies. Now that's not true! You don't need a medical degree in order to understand your own body. A lot of people don't know everything about their cars, but they can still use them and maintain them in good condition. The same is true of your body. If you don't fall prey to the "can't-understand myth," you can overcome the problem of the "no-control-of-health myth" even better. In other words, with sound knowledge and self-confidence, you don't *always* need a doctor.

You should remember one very important fact concerning doctors. Doctors, nurses — indeed, all of medicine — only help your body to help its self. That's the bottom line. Your body has the major part of the job in fixing a problem. If you get an infection, we give you an antibiotic (if we have one for that particular germ) to help kill the bacteria, and then with time your body can get rid of the rest of the infection. If you get appendicitis, a surgeon will remove the inflamed appendix, and then your body gets to work repairing itself. In other words, your body does it all (with a little help from its friends). Its major friend is you. *You must take care of yourself.* If you ignore problems, mis-treating yourself for a long time, you can throw away your body's reserves. Then one day you'll get a problem, and your body won't be able to respond. And that problem might overwhelm you. Remember, we only help.

Returning to doctors again, they're the ones who give out prescriptions for pills, which leads to another erroneous belief—"there's a pill for every ill." Wrong. If all I did was watch TV, and if I didn't know better while I was watching, I would probably believe this myth. Got a headache? Take a pill. Nose stuffed up? Take a pill. Constipated? Take a pill. Need anything at all fixed? What else? Take a pill.

If pushed, I'm sure that most of us would admit that there isn't a pill for every ill, but the belief is so widespread (and so easy to believe) that many knowledgeable people still hold to it. And what would be easier than being able to take a pill for anything that goes wrong. I fear that belief in this myth leads to complacency, as does the next one.

A great many people feel that any problem—even health—can be fixed, and fixed instantly at that. When confronted with the fact that "it ain't necessarily so," a number of people get angry. It's almost like the disappointment you feel when you learn that there is no Santa Claus. That anger doesn't help, and it often gets in the way of effective treatment of the problem. I see this happening all the time; it seems that belief in instantaneous correction of anything comes from both wishful thinking and the Big Mac syndrome. We wish that anything can be fixed so we don't have to worry about possible problems. As for the Big Mac syndrome, our modern society has become one of quick, almost instant gratification. "I want my Big Mac, and I want it now!" (And you quickly get it.) So, we can be complacent about things because we hold the myth of instant, every-problem-correction in the back of our minds. Complacent people don't concern themselves with the future, nor do people who believe in the Four Free's.

Forgive my cynicism, but I sometimes think that most people believe that life is pain-free, stress-free, trouble-free, and just plain *free*. Also, throw in the myth that "perfection is possible." Once again, when you believe those myths you can't easily accept the realities of health, namely that your body is not perfect; pain is occasionally going to happen (it's your body telling you something is wrong) as is stress; therefore, you have to actively help yourself. Those beliefs also encourage complacency and a lack of self-care and self-respect, although I think the final myth is the one that most fosters complacency—the INHTM belief.

The INHTM Syndrome: *It'll Never Happen To Me*. This is the root of all our self-disregard. Denial is a powerful force, and we all deny future possibilities at one time or another, some more than others. Why? Well, I think we use denial to prevent confrontation with our mortality. Life is a "package deal"—you're born and you must die. When you're young it's impossible to conceive of your death, but when you get older you become aware of your eventual end. Look around the edge of that wall of denial and you stare right at that ending, so you stay behind the wall, fully knowing what's on the other side. Since you're not constantly confronting that demise, you can deny it, so you can usually function without conscious awareness of it. To me, this seems to be an act of defiance.

We can believe these myths because modern medicine permits us to. Medicine is a double-edged sword—it cuts both ways. On one hand, modern medical care can treat many conditions, and we're learning how to take care of many more each year. That's the forward stroke of the sword. The back stroke is the problem. As we've become more and more aware of how good medicine can be, we've grown secure and complacent—we don't have to care for ourselves. In many instances, if we're not encouraged or even made to do something (in this case stay healthy), we won't do it. Especially when we're convinced of the fact, that whatever we do (or don't do) to ourselves can be fixed.

Here's an example of that attitude. Recently a man told me he didn't have to think about these things since he probably has a better chance of dying by being hit by a car while crossing the street. I wouldn't argue the point at that time, but later the flaw in his logic dawned on me. I'm sure that whenever he crosses the street he automatically checks both ways so he won't be hit. It's something he has done for years, ever since Mom and Dad let him cross alone. In other words, he looks ahead; he takes care of himself. Now, if we could just get him, and you, and everyone to do the same thing in most situations, we'd take better care of ourselves. But we don't do it.

So we hold onto our mysterious myths, and in the long run they interfere with good health. They make us complacent about the future. We lose the necessary sense of cause and effect—eat two extra chocolate chip cookies every day and you eat about 100 extra calories, which will give you 1 extra pound in 35 days and over 10 extra pounds in a year! Cause and effect. What you do now will certainly affect your health sometime in the future. Disregard those myths. Have some respect for yourself. Why not make your life a Well-Fit Life?

Well-Fit Tips

You can understand your body.
Respect yourself and have confidence in yourself.
How you treat yourself today will affect your future health.
You can influence your health — positively or negatively.

2

Killing Softly

Do you remember the Roberta Flack tune, "Killing Me Softly With His Song?" That phrase is very apt for our country—we are killing ourselves softly. We're doing things to ourselves that are killing us early, things that work slowly, quietly diminishing our life expectancy and quality of life. What things? Smoking, drinking, being fat, indulging in bad foods, inactivity, having too much stress, to name a few.

The question of human cost can be answered on two levels—the national picture and the personal tragedy.

First in money, everyone's bottom line. In 1980 the total costs for health care in the U.S. were somewhere around $240 billion, and the current guess is that those expenses will get up to $765 billion by 1990. Without doubt we're going to run out of money. Sums that high are going to affect our economy in the wrong way.

With respect to the economy, our businesses are having a great deal of financial trouble due to the poor health of their employees. Premature death is thought to cause a loss of about $19 billion, while illness alone contributes an additional $3 billion in losses. What about alcohol, our most readily available drug? Accident rates for a drinker are 2 to 4 times that for a non-drinker. The total cost of alcohol-related problems comes to about $5 billion. Up to 80% of adults in this country will have low back pain at one time or another, and losses from that problem are about $1 billion. Notice that all of the financial figures I gave are in *billions* of dollars. That word is used so often these days that we've grown accustomed to it, but few of us can really conceive of what a billion dollars is, not to mention the $200 *billion* American business spends each year on health insurance alone.

Enough about money. What about the number of people with these and other problems? About 1½ million people in this country will have a heart attack this year, and over half a million of them will die from it. Heart disease is our number one killer. Cancer is number two, while stroke and similar problems rank number three. Close to half a million people will die this year from cancer, with lung cancer leading the list. Of the more than 1½ million people who will have a stroke this year, close to 200,000 will not survive.

As for heart disease, almost 42 million people have some form of heart or blood vessel disease. High blood pressure, the silent killer that leads to heart attack, affects 15% of U.S. adults or over 30 million people. One of the major contributing factors to high blood pressure, of course, is obesity. And remember the low back problem that I mentioned above? One of the contributing factors to it is also obesity; some experts feel that close to 97 million people in this country are either overweight or obese. That's almost *half* of the population.

Now let me try to bring these problems home to you, because they will affect all of us. Don't ever think that you won't *ever* have any health problems! Random chance affects everyone, and our present lifestyles only increase the probabilities for the major diseases. They *can* happen to you. While you're reading about them, stop and think about yourself.

Some people say that we Americans can accept only three causes for death—auto accidents, heart attacks, and old age. Accidents rank number 4 on the list of causes of death for all ages combined, yet they are number 1 for young adults. The auto contributes the most accidents. Remember the last chapter's INHTM syndrome? I sometimes think that almost everyone chants "It'll Never Happen To Me" when getting into a car without using seat belts. But the same can't be said for those driving under the influence of alcohol. Drinking is involved in over half of fatal auto accidents.

I once took a survey of all the patients involved in auto accidents I saw during more than a year of working in the Emergency Department of a hospital in York, Pennsylvania: I found a total of two who had been wearing their seat belts. Two out of hundreds. Most of the non-wearers said, "I don't wear it because I don't want to be trapped in the car," or something similar. Also, many of those accident victims had been drinking. Drinking, driving, and no seat belts are commonly accepted. How about you?

Let's shift gears and look at heart attacks. Unless I miss my guess, I'm pretty sure that most of you reading this think you'll never have a heart attack. Don't be too sure. Or too smug. I remember one recent day at the hospital when four young people in their thirties arrived with chest pains. Two were false alarms, but one man had a massive heart attack, and a woman was having an angina attack (her heart was starved for oxygen, but it hadn't gotten to the heart attack stage when there is no oxygen at all). Several days later we got a call on the radio. A 34-year-old man had been playing basketball, when he began to feel bad. He sat down to rest. Shortly thereafter he just fell over — his heart had stopped (arrested). A cardiac arrest in a young person is something none of us wants to see, especially when there is no reason for it, as was the case with this young man. We worked for over two hours trying to bring him back, save his life, but nothing worked. An autopsy was done, and it was discovered that he had had a massive heart attack. So remember that such a thing can indeed happen to you, particularly if you don't take care of yourself.

I often think that we actively try to shorten our lives through abuse. The following is a short list of what I'm talking about: smoking, alcohol, obesity, rich and refined diet, inactivity, high blood pressure, stress, and auto accidents.

Unfortunately, many of you live lives that put almost (if not all) of those things together. Think about it. You probably can think of someone (maybe even yourself!) who is fat, smokes, drinks, over-eats, has a stressful life, doesn't take needed medication, and has not had a regular exercise activity for years. Throw in being male, and you have a real problem. Odds are that that person will not live a long life. He is speeding-up his body's degeneration.

The package deal of birth and death has varied time between the two events. Your body's organs are working at maximum efficiency during the mid-20's, but they slowly lose efficiency as the ensuing years pass. With age your body handles physical stress less well. If you care for yourself you can keep the degeneration at its normal pace; indeed, you might even be able to slow it down just a bit. Abuse yourself, and you will probably hasten your body's breakdown. You might significantly shorten your time between birth and death.

The degenerative changes that happen in your body are slow, but like compound interest, they produce big changes after the passage of years.

Ever seen a lung cripple? That's someone who has had emphysema (caused mainly by smoking) — he or she can barely get around without being short of breath. Believe me, shortness of breath is scary. Take a soda straw, put it in your mouth, and close your lips tightly around it. Pinch your nose closed. Now, take a brisk walk, breathing only through the straw. You'll find out very fast what someone with emphysema feels *all the time.* An emphysema patient who has a sudden worsening of the disease arrives in the Emergency Department with terror in his eyes. Real terror.

Or how about a heart cripple? Some people get chest pain just by taking a walk. Some even get pain sitting still. These people usually go on to have heart attacks.

There are fat cripples also. There comes a time when your body can't manage its fat if you gain too much. Such people can barely walk. As a matter of fact, they have trouble breathing at all. Charles Dickens described such a person, the fat boy in *Pickwick Papers.* Today a person who is so fat that he or she doesn't breathe very often is said to have pickwickian syndrome.

Most of you don't have problems as bad as those, but stop and think now. Do you smoke? Have you been going out and buying smoker's tooth polish and breath freshener? Ever thought about *really* stopping?

Have you bought a car with a tilt steering wheel lately, a steering wheel that can clear your expanding belly? What's more, have you been buying beltless trousers with expandable waists so that they aren't too tight when you sit down?

Do you agree with Joan Rivers that the only good thing about exercise is stopping? With that attitude, do you spend 5 to 10 minutes looking for a parking place next to the entrance, and then wait at the elevator for several minutes instead of walking up that one flight of stairs? Do you use an electric can opener or an electric tooth brush?

I could go on and on, but I'm sure you get my point. The old adage "use it or lose it" applies to your body. Your loss might be a premature end. What's more, your time until that end could be very difficult — your quality of life could become very poor.

An unnecessary early death is a tragedy. I'm sure that you don't want to contribute to your own early demise. So, stop "killing yourself softly." It's never too late to begin, and a better way of life is available — as you'll see in the next chapter.

Well-Fit Tips

> *Bad health costs good money.*
> *An early death due to self-abuse is a needless death.*
> *Don't accept your poor health — do something about it.*

3

Wellness

The secret to staying alive, more alive, is no secret at all—it's been well known for centuries. For example, several thousand years ago, the Yellow Emperor of China, Huang Ti, wrote of disease *prevention* and *prospective* medicine.

Prospective medicine is "looking ahead" medicine. If you keep those erroneous myths and those self-destructive behaviors of the last two chapters in mind, you can avoid falling prey to them. You can live a life of prevention, self-respect, and wellness.

Wellness is a fairly awkward word that has been around since the '50's. Back then, Halbert Dunn, M.D., wrote a book called *High Level Wellness*. Since then, many people have come to the conclusion that a wellness approach to life can be very beneficial. Before we look at those benefits and how to get them, let's talk about wellness and what it really means.

Most of you would put your health at the top of your list of priorities. We've known that fact for years. Unfortunately, in our country (and many others) there is a paradox—even though we are very concerned with our health all the time, we do nothing about it until it goes bad. Good health is something we just expect to have without any effort. In other words, many of us live lives that are just above the "illness level," and we become concerned with our health only when we drop below the illness threshold and get sick. Wellness is something more. It's health with few limitations.

A person who lives a life of wellness, not one just above the illness level, receives many benefits. He or she has a higher quality of life. They can do what they want to. They aren't limited by their disabilities, their fat, their inactivity, their marginal health. Sure, such people also get sick. You can't eliminate fate or chance. But a "wellness person" often weathers the storm of that illness with fewer problems.

Wellness increases your chances of having a long life expectancy. Do you know the difference between life span and life expectancy? *Life span* is the length of time we humans can usually live barring any problems. Some researchers suggests that our life span might be around 100 years. On the other hand, *life expectancy* refers to the number of years each individual can expect to live. That time varies depending on your age and how well you take care of yourself.

At birth women have a life expectancy of 77 years (give or take a few), while men can expect to live 70 years after birth. The longer you live, the longer you can expect to live. For example, a 75-year-old has a life expectancy of about 10 years, a little less for men and a little more for women.

The important thing to remember is that you can drastically shorten your life expectancy through self-abuse. Smoking can shorten it by almost 10 years. Inactivity, stress, obesity, etc., all shorten what you can expect. I don't know anyone who wants a short life, but I do know many, many people who by virtue of their lifestyles are decreasing their years to live.

Life *style* is at the heart of the matter. Right now it seems that a bad, self-abusive lifestyle accounts for 57% of heart disease, 37% of cancer, 69% of auto accidents, and 70% of cirrhosis of the liver. Some experts feel that half of our deaths are due to unhealthy living. As a matter of fact, up to half of our total health care expenses are thought to be for problems that are potentially preventable. Half of $240 billion dollars is a lot of money! If we began to live lives of self-respect we could save a bunch of money, not to mention prevent many troubles.

So, a life of wellness can help you. To me the best way to achieve wellness is through fitness—physical and mental fitness. A Well-Fit life.

Your own Well-Fit way of life is possible. As you'll see in the following chapters, you can make yourself fit and well. You need to keep some things in mind in order to achieve your goals.

First and foremost, give yourself realistic goals. Don't expect to end up looking like Jane Fonda on the cover of her book, *Jane Fonda's Workout Book*. She's Jane Fonda, and you're you. Work on making yourself attractive in your own unique way. Don't expect instantaneous changes, quick weight drops. You became the way you are over *years*, and it'll take time to change for the better. Be realistic.

Second, don't get upset about failures. No one does everything perfectly. If something doesn't work, experiment, make changes. Accept the need for self-feedback. Listen to your body and trust yourself. Don't be afraid to do something just because you're afraid of failing. Learn.

Third, have fun. Don't become obsessed. Too much focus on improving your health can be unhealthy! Give yourself breaks, time-outs. Treat yourself occasionally, just do it in moderation. Involve your family, friends, and others in a friendly way. Don't become a pain in the neck for them or yourself. Enjoy yourself.

Fourth, and last, open your eyes. Look around you with a new viewpoint. You've probably been in a rut for years, just accepting the gradual changes of your body's degeneration. Don't passively accept things. Be active. Become your own best friend and helper. Remember, there are more involved than just yourself — you've got parents, perhaps a family, many friends. Improving your own health and quality of life will ultimately help them, too.

Someone once said that a life is greater than the sum of the parts of it, greater than your body, mind, and spirit. Wellness, fitness, self-respect, knowledge of the future all serve to expand your life. Use the Well-Fit Way and be alive, truely alive.

Well-Fit Tips

> *Wellness provides a longer life expectancy and a better quality of life.*
> *Well-Fit is wellness through fitness.*
> *Everyone can be Well-Fit.*

4

Your Condition

Back in the late 60's, Kenny Rogers sang a song entitled "Just Dropped In To See What Condition My Condition Was In" – and that's exactly what we're going to do now. We'll take a look at your present state of health, along with your height, weight, obesity, physical condition, and more. Get out your calculator, scale, tape measure, mirror, and let's get to work!

HEALTH HAZARD APPRAISAL

One of the recent advances in preventive medicine is the HHA, or Health Hazard Appraisal. A HHA allows you to get some idea about your current state of health, particularly if it is speeding up your eventual demise. That's right, the more sophisticated (and expensive) HHA's can actually give you your "health age," showing you your "age" with respect to your life expectancy. In other words, if you're not taking care of yourself, your "health age" might work out to be 50 while your real age is only 40. See the difference? You're speeding up your breakdown. Remember, eventual breakdown of your body is a part of life, but you don't want to hasten the process.

What are the factors these HHA's look at? Usually the risk factors examined include smoking habits, level of activity, richness of diet, stress, high blood pressure, amount of body fat, alcohol use, sex, and more. A combination of too much stress, too much dietary fat and

YOUR CONDITION   13

sugar, too much alcohol, smoking, obesity, and too little exercise can lead to real problems.

Now let's see how you stand in relation to these risks. The following is your Well-Fit Lifestyle Appraisal. It won't give you your "health age," but it should make you stop and think about your present lifestyle and how that way of life is affecting you.

In each of the following seven areas circle 0 points if you *Rarely* do the thing, 1 point if you *Sometimes* do the thing, and 2 points if you *Mostly* do the thing. Remember:

    Rarely   –0 points
    Sometimes–1 point
    Mostly   –2 points

Well-Fit Lifestyle Appraisal

Smoking
    I don't smoke   0   2
Alcohol, Drugs, Medications
    I don't drink or I have only 1 drink a day   0 1 2
    I don't use recreational drugs   0 1 2
    I take my medications as the label directs   0 1 2
Driving
    I don't drink and drive   0 1 2
    I use my car seat belt   0 1 2
Activity
    I exercise 3 to 4 times a week   0 1 2
Obesity
    I stay at my ideal weight   0 1 2
Diet
    I don't eat many sweets   0 1 2
    I don't eat much fat   0 1 2
    I don't use much salt   0 1 2
    I don't over-eat   0 1 2
    I eat a well-balanced, high fiber diet   0 1 2
Stress
    I take a daily time-out   0 1 2
    I handle stressful situations well   0 1 2

After you've circled one number in each of the 15 statements, add up all of your circled numbers and write it down below.

    Well-Fit Lifestyle Appraisal Total –_____

If your total is greater than 25, you're doing well for yourself and your health – you should be proud, and you should keep up the good work.

A score between 18 to 25 means that your lifestyle is good, OK, but it needs work. Dropping lower, a total in the range of 9 to 15 suggests that you need a fair amount of work, and you'd better get started, especially if you're at the lower end of that range of numbers. Those of you with scores of 5 and below are in trouble. Maybe things aren't too bad now, but you must think of the future and change your lifestyle. Respect your*self*.

To sum up:

Well-Fit Lifestyle Appraisal Scores — 26-30 Good
　　　　　　　　　　　　　　　　　　18-25　 OK
　　　　　　　　　　　　　　　　　　 6-17　 Need work
　　　　　　　　　　　　　　　　　　 0- 5　 Terrible

Before we leave the IIIA, I must stress one very important thing — of the 15 statements in those 7 areas, "I don't smoke" is the most important. Notice that it gets only two scores, a 2 or a zero. There's no middle ground. There's no compromise on smoking. You must *not* smoke if you want to be healthy.

YOUR BODY

Now that we've examined your lifestyle, let's look at your body. First, you should get some basic measurements — height, weight, and waist circumference.

Get someone to help you, and accurately measure your height in inches. I suggest that you back-up against a wall, getting your heels, back of your legs, buttocks, back, shoulders, and head against the wall. Stand up good and straight. Have your helper put a straight edge (ruler, book, etc.) on the top of your head, and put a small mark on the wall. Then you carefully measure from the floor to the mark. I know this sounds a bit silly, but I'm sure most of you haven't had your height accurately measured for some time.

Weigh yourself on a good scale. Don't worry about super accuracy. You don't need to run out and buy one of the tall scales you see in schools, clinics, and doctors' offices. Your present one will do. Stick with that one — you'll want to use the same scale each week for your weight.

Measure around your waist at the level of your belly button or navel. Use a mirror, keeping the tape horizontal all the way around.

Now, write down the results of your measurements in the spaces below and at the end of this chapter:

Height (in inches)　 — _____
Weight (in pounds) — _____
Waist (in inches)　 — _____

YOUR CONDITION

Next, we'll add two more measurements to give you your five basic parameters, four of which will change as you become Well-Fit. Our next two are resting heart rate and resting blood pressure.

Keep a wristwatch or clock by your bed for the next few days. Each morning for about three days take your pulse or heart rate shortly after you wake up and before you start moving around. Average the three values, and you've got your resting heart rate. By the way, for those of you who have never taken your own pulse, don't get concerned – it's very easy. Place the index and middle fingers of one hand on the wrist of your other arm, just below your thumb. Check the accompanying picture to make sure you have the right spot. Feel that

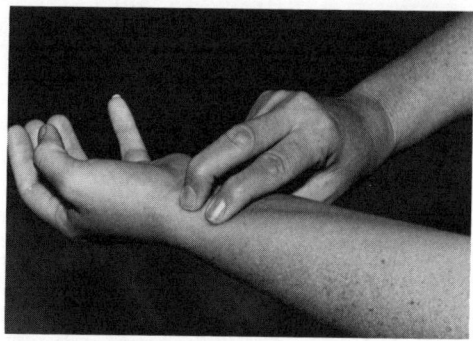

Fig. 4:1. Taking your pulse. The radial artery can be felt on the wrist. Place the index and middle fingers of one hand on the wrist area at the base of the thumb of your other arm as shown. You should be able to feel the beat of your heart. Count the beats for 6 seconds, and multiply that number by 10 to find your 1-minute heart rate.

throb against your fingers? That's your heart beating. Each throb you feel is one squeeze of your heart. Count the beats for 60 seconds. That's your resting heart rate. The normal for women is between 70 and 80, while the male norm is between 60 and 70.

Unfortunately, getting your resting blood pressure is not so easy. You'll probably need to have it taken by a nurse or doctor, but there are some self-measurement units on the market that you can try. I take my own blood pressure. It's really not hard. By the way, your local American Heart Association probably has a free class you could attend to learn how to do it. Check the white pages of your telephone book.

If getting your blood pressure is difficult, you can make this measurement optional, but if you haven't had it taken for some time, especially if you or your family have a history of high blood pressure, you might want to get it checked. If the value is 140/90, or 160/90 for those of you over the age of 50, then you have high blood pressure if it's elevated on 3 different days. See your doctor if you discover that you have the problem.

Write down your resting heart rate and blood pressure below and at the end of this chapter:

Resting Heart Rate – _____   Resting Blood Pressure – _____

All of these basic measurements except height should go down as you become Well-Fit. These are your starting points, so you'll refer to them to see how you're doing.

OBESITY

Many of you might be wondering if you're fat, or obese. Obesity means that you have too much fat, so much so that you're at risk for health problems like heart disease, diabetes, high blood pressure, and more. There's a quick way to see where you stand — it's called the BMI, or Body Mass Index — and you can quickly calculate yours with your pocket calculator.

Before we do it, I must explain something for you. This BMI is fairly accurate only if you're not a long-term weight lifter. The assumption is that you're fairly inactive. A weight-lifter can be overweight, meaning weigh more than the usual for his or her height, yet not be obese because his or her amount of fat is normal or even low. With that in mind, let's do some quick calculations.

The BMI is your weight in kilograms divided by the square of your height in meters. Don't panic. I'll lead you through this step-by-step.

Take your weight in pounds and divide that figure by 2.2, and you'll have your weight in kilograms (see equation 1 below). Next, multiply your height in inches by 2.54 and then divide by 100. That'll give you your height in meters (see equation 2 below). Multiply your height in meters by your height in meters, or square it (see equation 3 below). Now divide your weight in kilograms by the square of your height in meters and you'll have it — your BMI (see equation 4 below).

1) Weight in pounds ÷ 2.2 = _____

2) $\dfrac{\text{Height in inches} \times 2.54}{100}$ = _____

3) Height in meters × height in meters = _____

4) $\dfrac{\text{A} - \text{Weight in Kilograms}}{\text{B} - \text{Height in meters squared}}$ _____ = _____ BMI

Got that? If your BMI is greater than 30, you're obese. You have a health problem. What's more, if that BMI is greater than 40, you're very obese and you have a major problem to take care of in order to become healthy. All of you who have those high BMI figures should begin a weight-loss, fitness program slowly and carefully, checking with your doctor. But don't give up. You can become Well-Fit.

FITNESS

You might want to get some idea about your current state of exercise fitness. A good way to find out would be a stress test, and I encourage all of you over the age of 35 (particularly men) who have not been regularly active for some time to look into getting such a test. If you fit into that category, please read the next chapter carefully.

For you others, the Cooper 12-Minute Test can give you an estimate of your current fitness. This test was developed by Dr. Kenneth Cooper, the doctor who made *aerobics* a household word. On a measured course, perhaps a track, run as hard and as far as you can for 12 minutes. The distance you cover will give you your level of fitness. You must understand that this is a maximal test. It's hard to do, and it puts a strain on you. That's why I don't suggest that you do it unless you're a young, active person. For the exact levels of fitness, I'll refer you to Dr. Cooper's many books, including *Aerobics, Aerobics for Women, The Aerobics Way,* and others.

COMPREHENSIVE APPRAISAL

A complete, comprehensive appraisal of your current condition would include a detailed medical history, complete physical examination, resting electrocardiogram, lung tests, a stress test, and certain blood tests including blood counts and cholesterol/triglyceride levels. Such an examination could include more, so if you're concerned, you might want to look into this. Check with your doctor. Also, a number of fitness or wellness centers have opened in various communities; centers that offer such comprehensive exams under one roof. Check around in your community or with friends, relatives, etc., if you're interested. Whatever your condition, don't despair. You can help yourself.

Well-Fit Tips

> *Obesity can give you health problems.*
> *Weight, waist, resting heart rate and blood pressure all reduce with fitness.*

Initial Measurements—

Well-Fit Lifestyle Appraisal – ____   Resting Heart Rate   – ____
Height   – ____   Resting Blood Pressure – ____
Weight   – ____   BMI   – ____
Waist   – ____

5

Look Before Leaping

As with almost anything in life, you must look before you leap into an active fitness program. Severe diets can cause health problems, sometimes even death (those "Last Chance" liquid protein diets did a number of people in). Heavy exercise is also a bit risky, especially if you have some risk factors that you ignore or don't know about. Doing too much too soon can cause trouble. So let's talk about the risk factors and guidelines for beginning an exercise program.

The first risk factor we'll look at is the most important – so important that all of the next chapter is about this problem: *Smoking.* If you smoke you have what I consider to be the worst risk factor of all. There's no getting around it – *you must stop smoking.* Smoking and a Well-Fit life can *not* go together.

High blood pressure, or *hypertension,* is a big risk factor. This is a medical problem that affects up to 15% of the adults in this country, especially blacks; many people with the disease don't even know they have it. High blood pressure is called "the silent killer." If it goes undetected and untreated for too long, it can cause kidney disease, heart disease, strokes, and more. As I told you in the last chapter, if your blood pressure is 140/90 (160/90 if you're 50 years old or older), you have hypertension.

Like high blood pressure, abnormally high amounts of *fats in the blood* are an unseen risk factor. Some people have this problem because of their heritage—they were born with it. Unfortunately, our high-fat diets also add to the problem. There is a laboratory blood test called a Lipid Profile that can show you if you have this disease. More about dietary fat and fats in the blood in Chapter 10.

There, you now know the three most important heart disease risk factors. A brief list of others would include known heart disease, previous heart attack, "hardening of the arteries," diabetes, strong family history of heart disease, obesity, too much constant stress, long-term inactivity, and being male. That's right, gentlemen, you have a greater risk of heart disease than women have.

When you were reading that list of other risk factors above, did you notice anatomy abnormalities? Sometimes you can be born with a variation in your anatomy or body structure that can be a potential problem. Often you're not aware of that variation. Indeed, you might live your whole life without any problems, but that change could suddenly make itself known. In several studies on sudden cardiac death with exercise, the vast majority of those under the age of 30 who died were found to have some heart structural abnormality. If you've become very dizzy, short of breath, felt many abnormal heart beats, or fainted while exercising, you should get a comprehensive medical check-up no matter what your age, sex, or risk factors.

Speaking of age, the number of years you've been around counts as a risk factor. In our inactive, "I don't want to do anything physical" society, we seem to break down pretty fast. Studies have shown that 35 years of age is the cross-over age.

Who can exercise? The American College of Sports Medicine answers that question with a classification list. At the top of the list is the symptom-free, regularly active person of any age without heart disease or risk factors. At the bottom of the list are those people who must not exercise at all (known heart disease, etc.).

The bottom line is the following—if you're over 35 years old and you've done no regular physical activity for years, get a check-up. Those of you under the age of 35 who have been inactive but do not have any heart disease or risk factors probably can begin an exercise program without a check-up, but use common sense—go slowly. Those of you of any age with risk factors or known heart disease need to get a medical clearance before beginning. The usual test is a monitored stress test on a treadmill or stationary bicycle, and that test can clear you for exercise while it gives you your exercise tolerance.

Is exercise safe? I'm sure that many of you are now asking yourselves that very question. My answer is *yes,* if you use your head. Get a medical check-up if you need one. Don't hurt youself.

Well-Fit Tips

If you need one, get a medical check-up before exercising. Exercise is safe if done correctly and in moderation.

Resources

American College of Sports Medicine: *Guidelines for Graded Exercise Testing and Exercise Prescription,* 2nd Edition. Philadelphia, Lea & Febiger, 1980.
Table 1 on page 3 lists the Exercise Classifications, while Table 2 on page 5 presents the Major Risk Factors. Also, Table 3 on pages 12-13 gives the problems that prevent exercise. This is a book for medical people, but it does provide a concise summary of risks, exercise tests, and exercise prescriptions. If you're interested in reading source material, it might be for you.

6

Smoking

If you don't smoke you don't need to read this chapter. Congratulations, you're well on your way to your Well-Fit life. If you do smoke, read on – we're going to take a look at what smoking does to your body, and some ways to break this habit. Actually, this could be the briefest chapter in the book, a chapter just two sentences long. If you smoke, stop. If you don't smoke, don't start.

I have yet to understand why people start smoking, but I can understand why they continue with it. Smoking is both a habit and an addiction. It's a psychological habit – you're used to it, and you need to do it. More important, your body is physically addicted to the drug *nicotine* contained in the smoke. It's hard to give up something that grips both your mind and your body.

In regard to your body, have you ever wondered what smoking actually does to you? Let's look at the immediate changes due to the habit first, and then we'll discuss the long-term effects.

When you light up a cigarette and inhale, you breathe in a number of things – nicotine, carbon monoxide, harmful gases, tars, and cancer-causing agents. The list is quite long. These things cause a prompt increase in the resistance to air flow throughout your lungs. In other words, it's harder to get the air in and out. That can be a real problem, especially when you consider that you need to breathe faster, both while you're smoking and for some time after you finish, because the amount of oxygen in your blood is lowered. Your heart rate and blood pressure also jump up. These things can cause substantial problems for someone whose lungs and heart are not well. As bad as these immediate effects are, they pale in light of the long-term problems from smoking.

A long-time smoker usually suffers from chronic cough and sputum production, along with breathlessness (not to mention stained fingers and teeth and bad breath). Smoking causes chronic bronchitis and emphysema. Chronic *bronchitis* is a prolonged inflammation of the air passages in the lungs, while *emphysema* is the actual destruction of lung tissue—lose too much tissue and you can't get enough oxygen into or carbon dioxide out of your blood. You're in real trouble. A lung cripple is a terrible thing to see.

Cancer is the number two killer of men and women: Smoking causes up to 85% of all lung cancers. Among the many cancer-producing elements in cigarette smoke are polycyclic aromatic hydrocarbons (PAH's). In your lungs PAH's can be changed into harmless wastes, or they can become carcinogens (cancer-producing agents). They have been called "ultimate carcinogens" because of their ability to cause tumors. By the way, besides being in cigarette and marijuana smoke, PAH's are also found in coal soot, diesel exhaust, and charcoal-broiled steaks. Besides these substances, the smoker inhales radioactive particles. If these things are in the lungs for long enough, the lung cells change, and cancer can result. And if that's not bad enough, the *nonsmoking family members of a smoker have been found to have higher rates of lung cancer.*

Heart disease and smoking are strongly linked. As a matter of fact, smoking is thought to contribute to one-third of all deaths due to heart disease. Add risk factors such as high blood pressure, high fats in the blood, and others, and you have real danger. Women taking birth control pills who smoke are included in this group.

Speaking of women, pregnancy and smoking don't mix. Pregnant women who smoke have higher occurrences of spontaneous abortions and premature births. Children of such mothers appear to have greater chances of growth and mental problems. Switching to men, smoking seems to cause some infertility by decreasing sperm movement, and cigarette use may cause impotence.

These are all health problems. What about the costs of these conditions? A total of at least $13 billion is spent each year on the medical expenses directly caused by smoking, and $25 billion is lost annually due to decreased work productivity. If that's not enough, we lose $180 million each year from the costs of fires started by cigarettes.

With all of these bad effects of smoking, you might ask why do 37% of the men and 29% of the women in this country smoke? The answer to that question is very complex.

A recent survey done by a UCLA psychologist found that 92% of the smokers he questioned relied on smoking for relaxation as well as a way to get the nicotine they needed. Using cigarettes for relaxation is a contradiction, because smoking doesn't relax you—it stimulates your sympathetic nervous system resulting in increased levels of adrenalin, and increased heart rate and blood pressure—an increase in "tension." That's the opposite of relaxation. Also, smokers are addicted to that nicotine, so if they stop smoking they go through withdrawal, getting headaches, shakes, irritability, and more.

Nicotine satisfies their addiction needs, but what about their habit needs? Over 60% of the smokers in the survey we just talked about said they also smoked "in order to keep their hands busy." They need the process of smoking—taking out the cigarettes, lighting up, etc. These habits are often triggered by cues such as eating, drinking coffee or alcohol, and so on.

Given these addiction and habit needs, it's not surprising why smokers find it hard to stop. Difficult or not, anyone who smokes *must* and *can* quit. The obvious question is how?

The most important thing about quitting is believing in yourself. You have to want to quit. A real need to stop is often based on two things—an understanding of the health problems of smoking, and (this is very important) a deep realization that those health problems can happen to *you*. Most of us deny such things, but believe me, those health problems can and will happen to you if you smoke.

Once you really want to quit the habit, you have to believe that you can. Yes, anyone can quit smoking. You might need help, and it'll probably be a struggle, but you can do it. Have faith in yourself. Also, there are some things that you can do to help.

Write down the time, location, circumstances, and your emotions on a record sheet wrapped around your cigarette pack every time you light up. I know that this will probably be a real pain, but it'll help you learn the cues that prompt you to smoke. Once you know those cues, avoid them. Substitute something else such as exercise or meditation. Enlist the help of your spouse, loved ones, and friends. If you do relapse, don't panic. Tell yourself that a small mistake won't hurt—you'll still accomplish your goal of quitting.

If you want and need group help, check into the various organizations that offer stop-smoking classes. There are a number in most communities. (See the list of resources at the end of this chapter.) Remember, everyone is different. Some of you will be able to quit alone, while others of you will need group help. Also, don't be seduced by those numerous cigarette ads you see almost everywhere. They push the incorrect notion that health and smoking can go together.

Look at the ads carefully. Every person in them is young, slender, and healthy. What's more, the majority of the models are not actually smoking. So don't be fooled. The decision to smoke is yours alone. It's not the decision of the tobacco industry that pays Madison Avenue 1 billion dollars a year to get you to smoke.

Finally, and most important, don't give up. You can do it. You *can* quit. That will be your greatest Well-Fit accomplishment, something you can be proud of for the rest of your life.

Well-Fit Tips

> *Smoking kills you early, and it makes you sick on the way.*
> *If you smoke, you* must *stop.*
> *If you don't smoke, don't* ever *start.*
> *A Well-Fit Life is a life without smoking.*

Resources

> For group classes or other help you may want to contact:
> American Cancer Society
> American Heart Association
> American Lung Association
> SmokEnders International
> Schick Centers for the Control of Smoking

7

Alcohol And Other Drugs

Let's move from nicotine to other drugs, beginning with the most commonly used and probably oldest known drug – alcohol. Some people estimate that up to one-third of adults in the U.S. drink more than 4 drinks each week, and one-third of those frequent drinkers can be called alcoholics. That's about 10 million men and women. They're mostly in the 35–55 age range, and there are many more men than women. Contrary to popular belief, only about 3%–5% of these problem drinkers fit the "bum" stereotype.

What does this drug do to you? Chronic drinkers can get cirrhosis of the liver, swelling of the belly from fluid, depressions and confusion, sexual problems, eye problems, pancreatitis (inflammation of the pancreas), nerve disorders, and more. Alcohol also contributes to heart disease and high blood pressure. Alcoholic mothers who drink through pregnancy can give their children the fetal alcohol syndrome – birth defects such as mental retardation, growth problems, and abnormalities of the face.

Alcoholic problems cost money. In 1975 the total cost of U.S. alcohol abuse and alcoholism was about $43 billion. What's more, alcohol is involved in more than half of fatal auto accidents, 64% of killings, 41% of assaults, 34% of rapes, 30% of suicides, and most unfortunately, 60% of all child abuse.

Given all these problems, it's obvious that a Well-Fit Life doesn't include excessive alcohol use! Notice that I said *excessive* use. Unlike smoking, you can drink a little alcohol and still be Well-Fit. How much is a little? No more than one ounce a day. In other words, you can have *one* mixed drink, *one* beer, or *one* glass of wine. Please remember my emphasis on *one* — you can drink one drink a day, not the whole six pack of beer or bottle of wine or whiskey.

For those of you who are alcoholic, you can't have any alcohol at all after you stop drinking. I'm sure you realize that fact, and I'm also sure you know how difficult it is to stop. The best known and largest organization for helping people to stop drinking is, of course, Alcoholics Anonymous. I strongly suggest that you contact this organization for help, either for yourself or for a loved one or friend.

CAFFEINE

Did you know that the people of this planet drink more than 4 million tons of coffee every year? That's a lot of coffee — and a lot of caffeine. Besides being in coffee, caffeine (and similar substances) is also found in tea, soft drinks, chocolate, and many over-the-counter and prescription drugs. A typical cup of coffee contains about 80 milligrams of the drug.

Caffeine and its related compounds (they're all called methylxanthines) are stimulants. They've been used as stimulants for thousands of years — the Buddhist meditators of long ago used strong tea in order to stay awake — and we continue to use them in the same way.

Caffeine does a variety of things to you. It stimulates your brain, combating drowsiness and fatigue. Your heart is stimulated, so it beats faster and increases its output. That increased output of blood goes through blood vessels that open up as a result of caffeine. The drug also relaxes the air passages in your lungs to some extent, while it increases the strength of contraction of your muscles. Caffeine makes your kidneys work harder, so you urinate more. Overall, your metabolism goes up.

Caffeine obviously does many things to you, but is it safe? Some experts now think that the drug can cause or aggravate some health problems, among them birth defects. The jury is still out on the matter. Even so, I feel that you should use caffeine moderately, perhaps drinking only 2 cups of coffee a day. Pregnant women should avoid the drug altogether (as they should most other drugs).

DIET PILLS

A while ago the Food and Drug Administration approved a drug called phenylpropanolamine for use in diet pills. I'm sure you've seen those pills in the drugstore—there are many different brands, over 70 as a matter of fact. The drug is also used in nasal decongestant pills, so it's fairly common.

Besides clearing your nose, phenylpropanolamine stimulates your brain, suppresses your appetite, and a few other things. Unfortunately, this drug also causes problems. Some people taking it have experienced high blood pressure, muscle damage, acute kidney failure, and even the symptoms of "speed" overdose. Phenylpropanolamine is not a harmless drug.

I strongly suggest that you *not* take any of those diet pills. If you follow the guidelines of this book, you'll lose weight without them.

RECREATIONAL DRUGS

Alcohol is a "recreational" drug. I suppose it's much more accepted because of the length of time we humans have been using it, but these newer drugs are not so accepted, and most of them appear to cause some fairly significant side effects. Avoid them.

MEDICATIONS

If you take medications, either over-the-counter or prescription drugs, take them as directed by your doctor and only when you need them. Remember, incorrect use of drugs can be harmful. Don't become dependent on pills (except for illnesses that really need them)—there's not a pill for every ill.

Treat drugs with respect, all drugs. Use them wisely and cautiously. A Well-Fit Life does not depend on needless drugs.

Well-Fit Tips

> *Use alcohol moderately—only 1 ounce a day.*
> *Have at most only 2 cups of coffee or tea a day.*
> *Avoid recreational drugs.*
> *Take needed medications only as directed.*

8

Stress

There's been a great deal of talk about stress during the past few years, and for good reason. It seems that our modern lifestyles are full of stress, and constant stress does bad things to us. Before we talk about the effects of stress, let's look at stress itself and try to understand what it really is.

Stress is very difficult to define. One way of putting it is that "a stress" is anything you have to cope with, and that coping can be physical or psychological or both. Imagine that you're walking easily down a level road on a warm summer day. You've been walking at the same comfortable speed for a while, so everything (your breathing rate, heart rate, etc.) is stable. Then you come to a hill. That hill is a stress—in order to walk up the hill and down the other side your body will have to increase its energy output, its breathing rate, heart rate, etc. Therefore you'll have to cope with the stress (the hill). Obviously, it's not a bad stress, so you manage quite well with it, relaxing after you've gone up and down it, and you continue on. Then something changes. You hear noises from your left, and glancing to that side you suddenly spot a very angry, very large bull charging right at you. Talk about a stress! To cope you can either fight like hell or run like hell. Since you haven't completed your bullfighting courses, and since you left your bullfighting cape at home, you opt to run like mad for the nearest tree. You successfully get up the tree before the bull successfully gets you, and then you're stuck up there, hanging on precariously in a very uncomfortable position while you stare eye to eye with your new acquaintance, the bull.

You had two stresses during your walk, a mild one (the hill), and a major one (the bull). Any stress forces you to cope so that you can reduce the strain of the stress, and that coping occurs in both your mind and body (obviously the two are linked together). We'll look at your body first.

Your body responds to stress with increased levels of adrenalin, increased blood pressure, breathing rate, heart rate, blood flow to your muscles, and sweating. You're ready to fight or run. What I've just described is the well-known "fight or flight" response first described by Dr. Walter B. Cannon of the Harvard Medical School. It's a primitive response, one that probably kept our ancestors alive back in the days when quite a number of "stressors" were out to eat them. We still have that response. Most of you have experienced it when you glanced into the rear view mirror while driving and noticed that flashing red light bearing down on you. Remember those feelings—sweaty palms, pounding heart, tension? You also felt the "let down" of the response when the trooper passed by you and you realized that he wasn't after you.

Psychological stress can also trigger your body's fight or flight response—that can be one of the ways you respond to a problem. Overall, your mind responds to stress with strain, and you can experience that strain in several ways: sadness, vigilance, and anxiety. The last one, anxiety, is the most common response. I'm sure many of you have felt anxious when you're under stress, and you've tried to reduce that uncomfortable feeling. As a matter of fact, a friend of mine, E. James Lieberman, M.D., a psychiatrist in Washington, D.C., feels that anxiety is the number 1 emotion that most of us try to avoid or reduce if we have it. We cope with anxiety in various ways, usually using one of the five most common methods of coping with major life stresses: information gathering, group affiliation, religious belief, denial, and optimism. All of us use our own technique. One very important characteristic of successful coping is getting a sense of control. Many people manage things much better if they know that they can control the situation.

Notice that I emphasized that people want to reduce anxiety. A reduction in anxiety produces a sense of relief, a relaxation. In the same way the fight or flight response also needs a period of relaxation after it's been triggered. Unfortunately, in our modern, stressful times we often don't get that relaxation, and that's one of the main reasons why constant stress is harmful.

HARMFUL STRESS

Constant stress that keeps triggering the fight or flight response doesn't give your body the chance to relax or recover. Your levels of adrenalin, blood pressure, and so on stay up for long periods of time. Keep things going too fast for too long and your body suffers—this is thought to be one of the reasons for high blood pressure, heart disease, and strokes.

What we're talking about is long-term stress that puts long-term strains on you and your body. Stresses such as family problems, job problems, money woes, and the like all take their toll on you. Eventually your body can't continue to cope, and you get sick. What's interesting about this is that people have different ways of getting sick—some get heart disease, some strokes, some cancer. This is fairly new information, but we've known for some time that there are some different personality types. Remember Type A and Type B people?

In 1974 Doctors Meyer Friedman and Ray H. Rosenman published a book entitled *Type A Behavior And Your Heart*. A Type A person is more likely to get heart disease than a Type B. The former is compulsive, over-achieving, always trying to do more and more, attempting to do too much in too little time. I'm sure that you've known such a person (maybe you're one yourself). On the other hand, a Type B person is more "laid back," self-confident, and able to handle things without too much strain.

These personality types point out something very important—your *appraisal* of a stress determines how you will react to it, and your personality influences that appraisal. Something very stressful to one person might not be a problem at all for someone else. If you're upset or anxious you might feel more strain in a stressful situation.

So it's obvious that stress can hurt you, and that you could help yourself a great deal if you could improve your ways of handling it. A Well-Fit Life can reduce your anxiety, improve your coping abilities, and give your body the capability to successfully deal with problems. We'll talk about how to accomplish those things in the next chapter, but first let's look at stress a little more.

You probably think stress is only caused by bad things. Think again. Good things also stress you. The famous Home-Rahe Life Stress Scale lists both bad and good things. Of course, divorce, death, loss of job and similar things are included, but you'll also find there getting a job, marriage, buying a house, and other "good" things. Remember, stresses are things you must cope with, and good things also force you to cope, as do things such as unfamiliar situations, airplane trips, noise, and more. By the way, noise is a real stress. Those of you who are using those lightweight stereo earphone radios and cassette players should be very careful. Besides over-stressing yourself, you can permanently damage your hearing if you turn the volume up too much.

We now know about bad stress, so let's turn to Well-Fit stress in the next chapter.

Well-Fit Tips

> *Stress comes from many things, things you must cope with.*
> *Too much stress for too long is harmful to you.*

Resources

> Selye, H. *The Stress of Life* (Revised Edition). New York, McGraw-Hill Co., 1976.
> Doctor Selye was the pioneer researcher in stress and its effects. This is a classic book about the problem.

> Friedman, M. and Rosenman, R.H. *Type A Behavior And Your Heart.* Greenwich, Fawcett Books, 1974.
> This is also a classic book. It presents evidence that personality types influence health.

9

Well-Fit Stress

Stress and anxiety are necessary parts of life. The anxiety of pre-competition often helps an athlete do well, as does the pre-opening jitters of an actor. My friend Dr. Jim Lieberman, whom I mentioned in the last chapter, often says that anxiety is the "cutting-edge of change."

Given that stress is important, but realizing that too much of it can be harmful, what can you do to have Well-Fit Stress? Several things, actually.

I suggest that you spend a week keeping a log book on the things that stress or bother you. Write down the time, day, situation, and the feelings you had about the matter (you'll get very used to such logs or diaries). At the end of the week, spend some time going over your entries, looking for ones that you could do something about. Sure, you can't easily solve job problems or financial difficulties, but you could do something about your family problems, health, and so on. For example, is there too much noise around the house? If the TV or stereo is always on, why not try to spend some time without them. Be creative – and considerate.

If you are a Type A person, work at changing yourself. It's never too late to do so. Read *Type A Behavior And Your Heart* (see *Resources* following Chapter 8), and follow the guidelines in it. You might need to enlist the help of your family, friends, or a professional counselor. Don't be embarrassed about asking for help. Believe in helping yourself . . . just becoming aware that you are Type A helps.

In the last chapter I stated that a very useful thing for coping with stress is a *sense of control.* In our hectic lives having more control would be very helpful. Time management can be beneficial. I'm not suggesting that we all become overly time-conscious, but rather that developing your own time management techniques can help to reduce stress, because you'll be able to accomplish more of the things you want. Use time wisely and productively.

TIME-OUTS

Speaking of time, to me a Well-Fit Life always includes a daily "time-out." A time-out is a period of time away from the daily routine which you set aside just for yourself. You must make sure that you schedule (if necessary) enough time during the day to have a time-out. A major pitfall with time-outs is that they often are the first things to be eliminated if the day gets too busy. That shouldn't happen. You have to convince yourself and your family that your time-out is *very* important, something that you need in order to be Well-Fit. Also, please respect the need for your family members to have their own time-outs. Everyone needs a daily "breather."

What should you do during your time-out? The answer is anything that allows your body to drop out of the fight or flight response into relaxation. Things such as reading, a pleasant hobby, exercise, or meditation help, and the last two—exercise and meditation—are the best ways to reverse the fight or flight response.

If you chose a hobby, pick one that you can really enjoy, not one that has a high frustration level for you. Don't get yourself even more worked-up during your time-out because you don't know how to do something. One example I can easily think of is the frustration I felt while learning to use the word processor I'm writing this book on (talk about a total sense of *lack* of control!).

Exercise is the best Well-Fit time-out. If it's done rationally and correctly, you can get away from things while you "burn-off" the fight or flight response and get fit in the process. At the end of your exercise period you should feel pleasantly fatigued but able to do it again. As we'll see when we cover exercise in detail later, I don't suggest that you exercise every day. On the days without exercise you can use your time-out period for that hobby, or you might want to add some form of meditation to your life.

Many Americans have negative feelings about meditation. Don't let those feelings stop you—*meditation is for everyone.* Remember what happens to you when you're reacting to stress? Increased levels of adrenalin, increased heart rate, blood pressure, and so on. Research has shown that meditation reverses those things—your adrenalin levels, breathing rate, heart rate, blood pressure all go down. You relax. You end the fight or flight response. That's marvelous stress management!

The easiest form of meditation that I've encountered is the Relaxation Response of Doctor Herbert Benson. Doctor Benson studied many people in his Harvard laboratory, and he found a very easy method of relaxing. It goes like this:

> Sit in a comfortable chair in a quiet room and relax. Close your eyes. Each time you breathe in and out, say the word *one* to yourself in your mind. Don't say it out loud. Breathe in and out—one. Breathe in and out—one. Do that for about 20 minutes. During that time, if thoughts come into your head, don't focus on them, instead just let them pass quietly away.

That's it. Simple isn't it? One more thing. Don't do this immediately after eating or exercising.

By the way, some people, particularly Kenneth R. Pelletier, Ph.D., a clinical psychologist at the University of California at Berkeley, feel that meditation makes you a more cohesive whole. After becoming adept at meditation, a form of focusing yourself, you are better able to have a unifying influence over your body's many systems. You handle stress better. Isn't that great? Besides being a form of stress management itself, meditation helps your *body* become more able to handle problems.

There are many other forms of meditation and relaxation, including progressive muscle relaxation, massage, Transcendental Meditation, and more. Any and all of them would help you overcome the fight or flight response during your time-out.

There you have it. Well-Fit Stress is stress that's helpful to you, and you now know some important ways to help yourself handle all stress. Later (in Chapter 17) I'll show you an easy way to include a time-out in your day and how to keep track of it.

Well-Fit Tips

> *Well-Fit Stress is a necessary part of life.*
> *Anxiety is the cutting-edge of change.*
> *Everyone needs a daily time-out.*
> *Exercise is the best time-out, and meditation comes in second.*

Resources

Selye, H. *Stress Without Distress.* New York, Signet, 1974.
Dr. Selye moves on from *The Stress of Life* in this book to present his ways to handle stress.

Pelletier, K.R. *Mind as Healer, Mind as Slayer.* New York, Dell Publishing Co., 1977.
Dr. Pelletier presents his views on how the mind influences health.

Benson, H. *The Relaxation Response.* New York, Avon, 1975.
In this book Dr. Benson clearly shows what his Relaxation Response is; why it works; and how to do it.

Carnegie, D. *How To Win Friends & Influence People.* New York, Pocket Books, 1981.
You're probably asking yourself — why does he have this book included in Well-Fit Stress resources? Because this is a tremendous book for helping you improve your relationships, thus reducing one area of stress. Don't overlook it.

Lakein, A. *How To Get Control Of Your Time And Your Life.* New York, Signet, 1973.
An excellent book to show you how to develop your own time management techniques.

10

Bad Food

Needless to say, we all like to eat. I don't think I've ever met anyone who doesn't enjoy eating—even those people suffering from anorexia nervosa are obsessed with food. Eating is enjoyable. Eating is fun. Eating is a time to visit with family and friends, a time to relax, discuss the happenings of the day, and plan for the future. Eating can lead to romance. Let's face it, food is great and eating it is even better! It's something we've always had to do, and the history of our love of food and eating is interesting.

Our early ancestors lived on insects, roots, nuts, and the like, but as they developed they became hunters, adding meat to their diets whenever they could get it. As civilization became more sophisticated we discovered how to use fire, and we eventually learned the basics of agriculture and the domestication of animals. From then on we had control over our food supply. This was a marvelous thing to develop, and as a result, we became creative with our food.

Over time we discovered alcohol, bread, and many other edibles. Food became a fascination, sometimes an obsession. Ancient societies developed their own unique tastes. For example, the Egyptians loved to get drunk. They, and the Romans who came later, perfected the "fine art" of vomiting periodically during great feasts in order to keep on eating (after all, your stomach can hold only so much). Speaking of Romans, an extreme case of conspicuous consumption occurred during the days of Julius Caesar—he is believed to have spent $25 million on food and wine for his friends (and horse) in one summer alone!

The Italians of the 15th century began using forks to eat, and they developed the techniques of enhancing the flavors of food with herbs, spices, as well as the cooking itself, instead of the usual method of preparation that overwhelmed flavors. The new Italian idea quickly spread around, especially to France.

Here in America, the native Indians were found to have many types of food—in the time of Columbus they had over 2000 different plant dishes. The European settlers of the New World brought their food fascination along with them, dedicating themselves to eating well, as we do now. But between then and now something extremely important happened that dramatically changed the way we eat—the Industrial Revolution. Modern methods of food preservation, transportation, processing, etc., were developed. We had entered the age of "bad food."

AMERICAN DIET

Not every food you eat today is bad for you. Indeed, almost every food is OK for you if it's eaten *in moderation*. Unfortunately, it seems that we Americans have a hard time with moderation, and the food that we're eating to excess creates problems over time. Let's look at what's happened to that food.

Time after time industrialization and affluence have changed the eating habits of many countries. The U.S. is no exception. Since the turn of this century we have increased our consumption of fats by more than 30% (and much of that is saturated fats), doubled our sugar intake while we've decreased our use of complex carbohydrates by more than 40%, lowered our amounts of dietary fiber by as much as 80%, and made our protein sources about 70% animal. What does that all mean?

PROTEIN FROM MEAT

Meat is a status symbol. Whenever a society gets more affluent, its consumption of red meat goes up, and that's not healthy. Red meat is very high in *fat*. You know what I mean—a well-marbled steak is highly prized. In Japan the process of getting well-marbled meat has been carried to the extreme. Ever heard of Kobe beef? In the area of Kobe, Japan, beef cattle are kept immobile in comfortable stalls where they receive daily body massages and diets of very rich food. Their body fat is greatly increased. The result is unbelievable. I've had a steak of Kobe beef. It was so marbled with fat and so tender that I could cut it with a knife using only minimal pressure. Unfortunately, the meat was also loaded with saturated fat.

We don't need all of that fat. What's more, we don't need all of the protein that we eat. In actuality, we probably need only about half of the Federal Drug Administration's Recommended Daily Allowance of protein, but we're a nation of protein addicts. So we eat meat like crazy and get too much fat. Of course, red meat does have its good qualities—it's a good source of protein, iron, vitamin B12, and so on, but it's high in fat. In addition, red meat is a very inefficient way to get protein. Instead of feeding grain to the cattle, we could eat it ourselves and eliminate the step of cattle production. The entire world would benefit.

FAT

We consume fat from more than red meat. We cook with it; use it on our food (salad oil, butter, etc.), and so on. Like sugar and salt, fat is hard to avoid. Our 31% increase in the amount of fat we eat has brought our fat habit up to between 40-45% of our total calories. Since many of us usually eat too many calories, we as a nation eat an astronomical amount of fat.

I'm mainly talking about saturated fat, solid fat; fat that melts when it's heated then re-solidifies when cooled; fat that is high in cholesterol. Animal fat. That's right, *animal* fat is mostly saturated fat in contrast to vegetable fats that are mostly polyunsaturated (also monounsaturated). For your interest, the terms "saturated" and "polyunsaturated" refer to the amount of hydrogen atoms on the fat molecules. Saturated fat is full of hydrogen atoms while polyunsaturated fat can accept 4 or more additional hydrogen atoms. Monosaturated fat lies between the other two. The problem with saturated fat is that it tends to increase the amount of cholesterol in your blood, and atherosclerosis ("hardening of the arteries") results.

SUGAR

Had any sugar lately? If you say no, you're probably wrong. Sugar is everywhere. I've even read that some cigarettes are laced with the stuff!

Sugar is *sucrose,* a molecule composed of glucose (blood sugar) and fructose (fruit sugar). That's all it is—a combination of two simple sugars. Talk about empty calories. Table sugar, or sucrose, gives you only calories, nothing else. So why do we eat it?

We become used to it early in our lives. Sweets, sweets, treats. Processed foods are high in sugar (and salt); you also find sugar in many medications. That's right, sucrose is used by drug manufacturers in many of their drugs. And what about soft drinks? We ought to call them sugar drinks.

How much sugar do we eat? Almost a quarter of our calories come from sugars, most of them being sucrose. Some people say that Americans get up to 60% of their total daily calories from the combination of sugar and fat.

SALT

Salt is another substance found in practically every food we eat. We're used to a salty taste. Ever noticed how many people salt their food before they even taste it? The salt I'm talking about is sodium chloride, NaCl. It doesn't give you any calories. Instead, salt is used by your body in its electrolyte balance: keeping potassium inside of the cells while sodium is outside of them creates a necessary weak electrical charge across the cell membranes. Salt is necessary, of course, but unfortunately, too much salt forces your body to retain fluid, one cause of high blood pressure.

FIBER

Fiber is non-digestible. It stays in your intestines adding bulk and retaining fluid. We've dropped our fiber consumption by almost 80% since the turn of the century. This has occurred mainly because our use of grains and vegetable products has steadily decreased as our foods have become more refined, while our use of such things as breads, etc., has gone down. Now we eat only about one-third of the amount of bread we ate in 1900.

REFINED AND PROCESSED FOODS

As a result of processing and refinement, our food has become high in calories and low in nutrients. To put that in another way, our food has high caloric density and low nutrient density. To get our needed nutrients we end up eating too many calories, or we don't get enough nutrients if we eat only the calories we need to maintain weight. What's more, our prepared foods allow us to stuff our mouths whenever we want to, sometimes all of the time. Our eating habits are shot to hell.

We eat out of appetite, our psychological needs, instead of out of hunger. We skip breakfast in the morning, or just have caffeine and sugar. Lunch is poor. As a result of this lack of nutrition, we really chow down at dinner, a meal that should be fairly light. We eat bad food, and we eat badly. Too much fat, sugar, salt, and caffeine go down our throats, along with too many calories, alcohol, and not enough fiber. The results? Bad health, disease and death.

HEALTH PROBLEMS

Too much fat intake can lead to heart disease – angina, heart attacks – and atherosclerosis. Twenty percent of men under the age of 60 will develop the problems of heart disease. Even more frightening is the fact that we're finding the changes of atherosclerosis in children! Those frequent visits to fast-food restaurants result in many meals that are very high in fat.

Speaking of dietary fat, high fat diets are now thought to contribute to colon and breast cancer, and the former problem, colon cancer, is also thought to be associated with high protein diets and low fiber diets.

How about one of our major medical problems – obesity? Obesity is connected with heart disease, high blood pressure, degenerative arthritis, strokes, and diabetes. Stuff your mouth too much, and you'll get fat. Get fat, and you'll get sick.

By the way, don't forget that sugar is the main cause of tooth decay which also leads to ill health.

There you have it. Once again, it's obvious that you are physically what you eat. So let's look at Well-Fit food, and see about eating right.

Well-Fit Tips

Eat poorly, and you'll have poor health.
You are physically what you eat.

11

Well-Fit Food

Now we'll turn from bad food to good food, Well-Fit food. Obviously, we have to eat to live, and "you are what you eat." I'd like to introduce a corollary to that old, well-known statement—you "eat" your health. Eat bad food (for long enough), and you'll have bad health. On the other hand, eating good food can help you maintain your good health. Of course, a true Well-Fit life includes more than just Well-Fit food, but more about that later.

GOOD NUTRITION

Good nutrition is very simple. It's based on just three principles: 1) common sense, 2) variety, and 3) moderation.

1) Use your common sense about what you eat. If you know that something is full of fat or sugar, eat less of it or none at all. In addition, eat foods that you like. Sit down with yourself and make a list of all the foods that you like. This will undoubtedly be a fairly long list, and when you have it prepared, move on to the next principle, variety.

2) I'm sure that most of you, if not all of you, have heard of the Basic Four Food Groups—cereals and breads; vegetables and fruits (and their juices); meats/fish/poultry; and milk and dairy products. You need to select your daily diet from these four groups. Get your list of favorite foods and separate them into their food groups. As you probably already know, your daily diet should have 4 servings from both cereals/breads and vegetables/fruits, and 2 servings from both meats

and dairy products. Use your favorite food/Food Group lists in selecting what to eat. That way you'll get the necessary variety, and you'll have on your menu each day foods that you like (*and that you'll eat*). We all know that variety is the spice of life, but I believe that many people suffer from food boredom—you're in a rut, eating the same foods over and over! Think about it. I can imagine that many of you have the same food routine, including your trips down the aisles of the grocery store. Often that boredom affects the way you eat, and you end up eating too much. To combat over-eating, remember the principle of moderation.

3) I can't over-stress the importance of this principle. We Americans don't practice that ancient advice, "moderation in all things" (derived from the Grecian "Golden Mean"). Our history has been based on just the opposite—unlimited land, unlimited wealth, unlimited opportunity—and that applies to our food. We have a seemingly unlimited quantity. But don't over-do it. (I know that's easy to say but hard to do.) Calories for energy are one of your basic nutrients, but too many leads to too much flab.

NUTRIENTS

Let's look at all of the nutrients your body needs to stay alive. Calories supply the energy needed for all of the internal processes that keep you going; any extra that you give yourself will be stored away as fat, that is, stored for a rainy day (and we don't have too many "rainy" days in this country). If you don't give your body enough calories* it will use its stored energy (and many of us have a great deal stored away), or itself. In other words, when you starve yourself, your body breaks itself down to get energy, so you can run into problems. I don't suggest that you drop below 1200 calories per day for men, or 1000 calories per day for women. If you do, you'll be in the starvation zone—and you want to lose just the fat, not muscles, etc.

Beside calories, your body needs the following nutrients: Protein (8 essential amino acids), Linoleic acid (the only essential fatty acid), Carbohydrates, Fat-soluble vitamins, Water-soluble vitamins, Minerals and trace elements, and Water.

---

*Let me quickly clear up something concerning calories. A calorie is the amount of energy needed to raise the temperature of 1 cubic centimeter of water 1° C.

WELL-FIT FOOD

Protein

Proteins are composed of amino acids, 8 of which your body can't make—the essential amino acids. These essential nutrients are listed below, along with the minimum daily requirement of each (in milligrams—mg) for a young adult male: Threonine 500 mg; Valine 800 mg; Methionine 1100 mg; Isoleucine 700 mg; Leucine 1100 mg; Phenylalanine 1100 mg; Lysine 800 mg; and Tryptophan 250 mg.

Notice that the required amounts differ. It's a characteristic of your body that it requires all of those 8 essential amino acids at the same time and in the same proportions as listed above. If, for example, you ate 7 of them in their proper proportions, but ate only *half* of the required amount of the remaining 8th one, *your body would only use half of the other 7*. Because of this fact, different foods have different biological values of protein. Milk and eggs stand at the top, followed by cereals, legumes (beans and peas), and then roots. In order to get the proper protein in a meal, you often have to depend on the principle of complementary proteins—by combining a protein that lacks some essential amino acids with another protein that has them in good quantity, you get a good biological value for your meal. Proteins are used as enzymes (which activate chemical reactions in the body), as parts of cell structures, as energy, and so on.

Fats

There is only one essential fatty acid—linoleic acid. You need only about 3 grams of it per day. Fats are used in cell structure, as hormones, as energy, and more. Some people state that in order for food to be palatable or eatable, it has to have a minimum of 40 grams of fat.

Carbohydrates

Carbohydrates are composed of sugars and starches. There are no essential ones. Their variety is enormous, and they are used by your body as your major energy source (along with fats), as well as for parts of your body structure, etc.

Vitamins, Minerals, Trace Elements

Vitamins, minerals, and trace elements are used by your body in various chemical reactions. Remember that you are essentially a large bundle of chemistry hard at work. These three groups of nutrients give you no calories, but they combine with various molecules, helping reactions take place. Another way of putting it is that they act as cofactors (or co-workers).

Here's a brief list of them: Fat-Soluble Vitamins: A, K, D, E. Water-Soluble Vitamins: Thiamin (B_1), Riboflavin (B_2), Niacin (B_3), Pyridoxine (B_6), Cobalamin (B_{12}), Folic Acid, Pantothenic Acid, Biotin, Ascorbic Acid (C). Minerals and Trace Elements: Calcium, Phosphorus, Magnesium, Potassium, Sodium, Chloride, Iron, Zinc, Sulfur, Iodine, Chromium, Manganese, Molybdenum.

Here is where this book differs from many other books on fitness—I'm not going to list the function and required amount of each vitamin, mineral, or trace element! Because, if you eat a Well-Fit diet—one that has good variety and the proper number of calories—you'll get all the vitamins and minerals you need. Also, you can create problems for yourself if you overdose on vitamins and minerals. If you're still worried about "getting enough," you could take *one* of the many daily vitamin and mineral capsules on the market—they won't hurt you. (More on vitamins in Chapter 24.)

Water

Your body is more than half water; you need to maintain your water balance. Trust your body—*drink when you're thirsty*.

WELL-FIT DIET

The Well-Fit diet is simple. You eat in moderation, getting a variety of the calories needed daily. The relative percentages of total intake each day of proteins/fats/carbohydrates are: Protein—15%—(high quality, complementary ones), Fats—30%—(no more than 1/3 saturated fats), and Carbohydrates—55%—(complex carbohydrates, 10% refined). In regard to carbohydrates, complex carbohydrates are foods such as pasta, potatoes, breads, etc. On the other hand, refined carbohydrates are candy, honey, etc. Concentrate on complex carbohydrates.

A diet of good variety and the proper number of calories will supply you with all of your nutrients. Remember to drink the proper amount of fluids. Your proper amount of fluids depends upon your thirst. Drink when you're thirsty, especially in hot weather. Keep your urine output going.

As you can see, the Well-Fit diet reduces the usual amounts of both proteins and fats, while it increases the amount of complex carbohydrates. The reduction in protein and fats (particularly saturated fats) will help to reduce your chances for getting those diseases we looked at in the previous chapter. Increasing your amounts of complex carbohydrates while reducing your refined sugar use will give you more fiber and nutrients (and less cavities in your teeth!). And yes, you can still have an occasional treat, such as a bit of candy, cake, or pie. Just stay within your calorie limits and make sure only 10% of your total carbohydrates are refined ones.

Overall, using the Well-Fit diet will help you in many ways. Remember, "you eat your health," so eat healthy. We'll look at an easy way to ensure that you're eating well in Chapter 18.

Well-Fit Tips

*You are what you eat.
Moderation in all things.
You eat your health.*

Resources

Brody, J.: *Jane Brody's Nutrition Book*. New York, W. W. Norton, 1981.
An excellent guide to the basics of nutrition. Written in a clear and very readable manner, this book can help you learn the things you need to know in order to give yourself good nutrition.

Lappe, F. M.: *Diet For A Small Planet*. New York, Ballantine Books, 1977.
This small book is written for vegetarians, but even if you don't want to give up meat, this volume provides a very clear explanation of the principle of complementary proteins.

Stare, F. J., and Aronson, V.: *Dear Dr. Stare: What Should I Eat?* Philadelphia, George F. Stickley Company, 1982.
This book is packed with good, solid nutrition information. In a question and answer format, Dr. Stare provides the answers for a balanced diet.

12

Fat

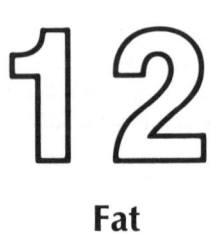

Believe it or not, we need body fat. It's our main storage area for energy, and it also acts as insulation and as a cushion for internal organs. The main problem with fat is that it is such a good place to store energy. Our bodies use it all the time.

Millions of years ago our ancient ancestors had a major problem — food was scarce. In that environment of "feast or famine," an energy storage system developed so that life could continue even when there was no food. We still have the same storage systems. As a matter of fact, the average, normal-weight adult male has about 140,000 calories of energy stored away. Given that such a person uses about 2300 calories a day, he could survive for approximately 60 days on just his stored fat alone!

Unfortunately, many of us have a great deal more than 140,000 calories stored away. Some statistical work has shown that close to 90 million Americans are overweight or obese — 30-40% of adult women, and 20-30% of adult men. That means that almost half of the adults in this country have too much fat on their bodies, and that leads to health problems. Before we talk about those health matters, it might be helpful for you to understand the difference between lean body mass and fat body mass.

LEAN BODY MASS VS. FAT BODY MASS

Your lean body mass includes everything other than fat — muscle, bone, brain, nervous system, internal organs, blood, etc. That's the stuff that keeps you going, keeps you alive. If you're set on losing weight, you want to lose excess fat, not lean body mass.

Your fat body mass is located in many places, but its primary location is beneath your skin, just above your muscles. This is called the subcutaneous (beneath the skin) layer. Here fat acts both as an energy depot and as insulation to help your body retain its heat. Fat also surrounds many of your internal organs, acting as a "cushion" as well as for energy storage. Finally, fat is located between muscles and in other little nooks and crannies.

Regular fat is also very active. As a matter of fact, the fats contained within your fat cells are always going in and out, with the result that all of your stored fat is recycled every 30 days. During that recycling you don't lose fat unless you give yourself less food and thus less energy to store, or increase your use of that stored energy through exercise.

HEALTH PROBLEMS

Too much fat, or being 20% over your ideal weight, leads to a number of health problems, including heart disease, diabetes, high blood pressure, degenerative arthritis, and more. At present, obesity is not considered a major health risk factor for heart disease directly, but it contributes to the problem in many ways. Often an obese person is extremely inactive, and eats a great many fatty foods. Sometimes such a person smokes. Obesity brings with it high blood pressure (a major heart disease risk factor) and diabetes (one of the direct causes of heart disease).

It seems that obesity causes high blood pressure because of an increase in the number of blood vessels your blood must pass through. It's been said that a pound of fat adds a mile of blood vessels to your body! In physiological terms, this massive increase in blood vessels leads to an increase in total peripheral resistance, or the resistance to blood flow. If this resistance goes up, it takes more pressure to move the blood through the blood vessels – the blood pressure goes up.

Diabetes is a damaging disease, and obesity can lead to one type of it – non-insulin-dependent diabetes. Insulin is the hormone that regulates your sugar or glucose metabolism. (A hormone is a chemical signal or trigger that tells cells to do things, and insulin tells cells to admit glucose, store fat, and more.) We now know that excess fat, or obesity, decreases the sensitivity of your cells to insulin. They don't get the message. To put it another way, obesity increases your insulin needs, and since your pancreas keeps putting out its usual amount of insulin, not increasing its output, you don't handle sugar well. Over time this sugar disorder causes problems.

Another problem related to obesity is degenerative arthritis. The increased weight associated with obesity acelerates the breakdown of your joints, particularly the hips, knees, and ankles. Those joints just aren't made to handle so much weight for too long.

GETTING OBESE

Given all of these problems, you might ask how people let themselves get obese. The answer lies in our storage systems. As I said, fats go in and out of your cells, usually in a balanced fashion. Take in too much energy (food), and you'll put in more fat than you take out. Over time the fat or flab that you have grows larger as the cells grow larger. Those cells can also grow in number, especially if you are obese in childhood. All of those cells sniff out any extra fats, etc., in your blood, grab them, and store them away. They're great at that job. (There are also some medical problems that cause obesity, but they're rare.)

So if you're obese, your job is to counteract the job of your fat cells. Take out more fat than they (the fat cells) can take in, and over time that flab will decrease in size. How far down do you want to go? We'll learn about that in the next chapter.

Well-Fit Tips

> *Obesity is having too much fat.*
> *Health problems occur when you're at least 20% over ideal weight.*

13

Well-Fit Weight

Look back to the Body Mass Index (BMI) that you calculated in Chapter 4. The BMI is based upon your height and weight, and as you know from the last chapter, your weight includes the weights of your lean body mass and fat body mass. I'm sure that you can see that someone who has been doing a great deal of weight lifting could be "overweight," meaning weigh too much for his or her height, yet be "underfat." The reverse can also be true. Someone can be at his or her normal weight and yet be "overfat." So, your ideal body weight (IBW) should conform both to the height/weight tables and to fat percentage.

FAT PERCENTAGE

Your fat percentage is the percent of your total body mass that is fat. Ideally, we should be a nation of normal fat percentage people, but we're not. The normal fat percentage for men is in the higher teens, 15-19% fat, while women should be about 20-25%, but the almost *90 million fat people* in this country are well above those percentages. Getting your fat percentage down to the ideal range takes time, exercise, and reduction in the amount of food you eat.

One word of caution. Bringing your fat percentage down too far can also cause health problems. Remember the unfortunate case of Karen Carpenter. The disease of anorexia nervosa — a psychiatric disorder in which the sufferer, usually a middle-class young woman, diets to extremes—is a problem that can cause death due to starvation. Everyone has a normal fat percentage, which varies a great deal from person to person, but when the percentage drops below 3%, it's usually considered pathologic (problem-causing). Athletes, particularly gymnasts, have low fat percentages—Olga Korbut was said to be 1½ percent fat when she won her gold medal at the Olympics! That's not normally found, and Ms. Korbut went down that low in order to be a good gymnast. You should try to stay in the normal range. When a woman drops down into the lower single digit fat percentages, she stops menstruating. Fertility suffers. Stay in the normal range, but don't go too far in the other direction—up.

IDEAL BODY WEIGHT

How can you figure out your Ideal Body Weight (IBW)? Get out your pencil and pocket calculator, and use the following formulas, knowing your height in inches:

Women — 100 lbs ± 5 lbs for every inch above/below 5 ft = IBW
Men — 110 lbs ± 5.5. lbs for every inch above/below 5 ft = IBW

Now let's figure out your IBW. Assume that you're higher than 5 feet tall (those of you less than 5 feet should subtract instead of add).

Inches above 5 ft _____(A)
Women — 100 + 5 × _____(A) = 100 + _____ = _____ IBW
Men — 110 + 5.5 × _____(A) = 110 + _____ = _____ IBW

That figure will put you in the ball park, and you'll be fairly close to the desired fat percentage, assuming that you are normally active.

Speaking of fat percentage, you might be curious about how much fat you have. There are several ways to determine body fat percentage, but the two easiest ones are under-water weighing and skin-fold measuring.

The former requires a pool of water, a scale, and a chair hung from that scale. You blow out all of the air in your lungs, and then you're totally immersed in the water. Then have your weight taken. Since fat floats more than lean body mass, the more fat you have, the less you weigh under water. Your fat percentage can then be calculated.

The latter method, skin-fold measuring, is less accurate than under-water weighing, but skin folds are easier to do. Using a pair of calibrated skin-fold calipers, measure the thickness of your skin in various places. Again, your fat percentage can then be calculated.

If you want to find out your fat percentage, check with your doctor, local hospital, local YMCA or gym, or at one of the Sportsmedicine Centers that are springing up across the country. As for reducing that fat percentage, you need exercise, so on to the next chapter.

Well-Fit Tips

> *Stay at your ideal weight.*
> *Don't put on too much fat.*

Weights

> Present Body Weight – _____
> Ideal Body Weight – _____
> Amount to Lose – _____

14

Exercise

According to my 1960 College Edition of *Webster's New World Dictionary*, the first definition of exercise is: "1. active use or operation; employment; . . . . ," while my 25th Edition of *Dorland's Medical Dictionary* defines exercise as "the performance of physical exertion for improvement of health. . . ." I want to add my own definition—*exercise is living*. We make active use of our muscles to stay alive—breathing, pumping blood, digesting food, etc.—in addition to using those muscles for physical exertion. Exercise is muscular work, and the only time you're *not* exercising or doing muscular work is when you're dead! Your old definition of exercise—breathing hard, heart beating fast, muscles working—is just the upper portion of the exercise or living scale, and like many other things, exercising at higher levels makes all of your muscular work more efficient. So throw away your old definition of exercise, and remember that you're exercising *all the time*.

WHAT EXERCISE DOES

Regular, rational, regulated exercise periods in which you get everything going at higher levels make changes in your body over time. We'll begin with the lungs and work down. I'm going to keep referring to aerobic exercise, which is continuous muscular work during which you get your body's metabolic rate up to high levels, but not to levels where you can't supply yourself enough oxygen. Aerobic exercise is muscular work with enough oxygen to continue working for a long period.

With long-term aerobic exercise your lungs become more efficient. It takes less muscular work to breathe. The muscles and structures of your chest move easier—in physiological terms, they become more "compliant." Also, the air passages of your lungs open up a little, so that there is less resistance to air flow in and out of your lungs. For someone who doesn't smoke and has no lung disease, the lungs are not the weak link in exercise.

Your heart also changes slowly with time and aerobic exercise. The main pumping chamber, the left ventricle, slowly enlarges, resulting in more blood being pumped with each beat of the heart. Again, in physiological terms, this means that the heart's stroke volume increases, and such an increase, coupled with an increase in what's known as "vagal stimulation" at rest, gives you a slower heart beat when resting. The lowest I've ever heard of is 26 beats per minute. I treated a female athlete last year who told me that her resting heart rate was that low at times. Also, the arteries of the heart dilate or enlarge somewhat; some studies have shown that careful exercise can even increase the number of blood vessels in a diseased heart.

Your heart pumps blood, and your blood volume increases with long-term exercise. That increased blood volume flows through greater numbers of blood vessels in your working muscles. Within those muscles the oxygen delivered by the blood is used more efficiently, because the energy-producing reactions that use glucose or fatty acids along with oxygen have more enzymes to work with.

The bottom line is that your aerobic capacity, or the amount of oxygen your body uses at full output per unit of time (usually a minute), goes up. This is a healthy change, and it's brought about by increases in the efficiency of both your oxygen delivery systems—lungs, heart, blood, blood vessels—and your oxygen use systems—muscles plus energy reactions within the muscles. In other words, your body is more ready for physical stress. It becomes used to an increase in breathing rate, heart rate, muscular movement, and so on.

BENEFITS OF EXERCISE

Chronic aerobic exercise, if done rationally, keeps your body well-tuned. If you suddenly have to do something that places physical demands on you, your body is prepared to do it. For example, shoveling snow won't kill you. Also, the increased metabolic or physical demands of an illness won't over-strain your body. You have more capacity to handle the stress, and to recover from it.

Speaking of stress, you'll recall that in Chapters 8 and 9 I talked about stress, and that in Chapter 9 I told you that exercise is a great stress management tool. Don't forget that fact. As long as you exercise *rationally*, not over-doing it, you'll come out ahead (and relaxed).

Exercise helps you to lose weight. It's especially effective in changing your fat body mass to lean body mass ratio, because it burns off calories (and fat) while it increases the size of your muscles or lean body mass. A combination of aerobic training and strength training (increasing the strength of your muscles) is most helpful. More on aerobic and strength training in Chapter 19.

You can also go a long way toward your goal of stopping smoking when you add an aerobic exercise program to your life. Many studies have shown that smoking and chronic exercise don't mix.

Finally, and perhaps most important, exercise is fun. It's an enjoyable way to learn more about your body and yourself; to gain fitness; and to have more control over your life. In the next chapter I'll show you the basics of Well-Fit exercise.

Don't have the attitude toward exercise that Joan Rivers talks about in one of her radio commercials for a diet soft drink—"the only good thing about exercise is stopping." Remember, exercise is *living*.

Well-Fit Tips

Exercise is living.
Exercise is fun.
Exercise improves your body.

15

Well-Fit Exercise

Now that you know what exercise is and what it does to you, it would be a good idea to talk about Well-Fit exercise, or rational exercise. Exercise can hurt you if done wrong (doing too much, too soon), so you need to know how to monitor what you're doing; your heart rate is the thing to keep track of while you exercise.

In Chapter 4 you learned how to take your own pulse or heart rate while at rest. Now you'll need to take it while you're exercising, but first you need to figure out your maximum heart rate.

As you grow older your body's capabilities decrease with the passage of time. Maximum heart rate is no exception. In other words, the fastest your heart can beat when you're exercising hard as you can declines with age. You can achieve your highest values when you're in your late teens (around 220 beats per minute). To figure out your predicted maximum heart rate, subtract your age in years from 220 like this:

$$HR(\text{Heart Rate})_{max} = 220 - \text{age}$$
$$= 220 - \underline{\hspace{1cm}} = \underline{\hspace{1cm}} (\text{per minute})$$

Figure it out now, but remember the figure because you'll need it later.

TRAINING ZONE

Now that you know your maximum heart rate, you can figure out your heart rate exercise training zone. That is, you can know the minimum and maximum rates you want your heart to beat while you're exercising. As you recall, your heart rate goes up when you exercise, and by knowing how fast you want your heart to beat, you'll exercise the Well-Fit way, the rational way.

The minimum level that you want to get your heart rate up to when you exercise is about 70% of your maximum heart rate. When you're exercising at that level you'll be giving your body a good training effect, a stimulus to change and adapt to the exercising, changing as described in the last chapter.

On the other hand, the maximum level that you want your heart rate to reach is about 85% of your maximum heart rate. If you go much higher than that you'll run out of oxygen. You'll have crossed the anaerobic (without oxygen) threshold. You'll hurt, and you'll have to stop exercising, something you don't want to do until your exercise period is over. So, let's figure out your training zone:

Highest Exercising HR:
$HR_{max} \times 0.85 =$ _____ $(HR_{max}) \times 0.85 =$ _____ (per minute)

Lowest Exercising HR:
$HR_{max} \times 0.70 =$ _____ $(HR_{max}) \times 0.70 =$ _____ (per minute)

You now know how hard to exercise.

Most people start out by exercising too hard. As a result, they hurt, and they quit. Remember, *rational* is the key word. Stay within the training heart rate zone, and you'll be exercising the Well-Fit way.

"LSD"

I've been asked many times why the training zone is important. When you exercise in the zone your body changes. Actually, you could get the same changes if you didn't exercise so hard, but you'd have to exercise for a number of hours a day. At lower levels of exercise you have to compensate for the loss of training intensity by using increased training durations. Long, easy training is often called Long Slow Distance (LSD) training. Unfortunately, to successfully use LSD training, you would have to exercise for a long, long time, something few of us can do in our hectic lives. We just don't have the time. A great deal of research has shown that shorter training periods can give your body good training stimuli if they are intense enough. Thus the training zone—it gives you sufficient intensity. In Chapter 19 I'll show you how many times a week you should exercise and what exercises to use. Anything that gets your heart rate up and holds it up for a while will do.

WELL-FIT EXERCISE

LOW RESTING HEART RATES

By the way, the formulas given above for figuring out your training zone assume that you have a normal resting heart rate (women—70, men—60). If your heart rate is a great deal lower than normal (10 beats per minute or more), you'll have to use a different formula for calculating your training zone; a formula that takes into account your low resting pulse. It goes like this:

Highest Exercising HR:
$[(HR_{max} - HR_{resting}) \times 0.85] + HR_{resting} =$ _____(per min)

Lowest Exercising HR:
$[(HR_{max} - HR_{resting}) \times 0.70] + HR_{resting} =$ _____(per min)

Some of you may naturally have low resting heart rates, while others of you may have lowered your resting rates through training, and yet another group of you may be taking medication that slows down your resting heart rates (usually drugs called beta blockers). If you fit into the slow resting heart rate category, please use the formulas just presented.

TAKING YOUR EXERCISE HR

Finally, a word about taking your exercising heart rate. I suggest that you stop your exercising activity for 6 seconds; count your pulse rate during that period; and then multiply the result by 10 to give you an estimate of your one-minute exercising rate. Stopping for much longer than 6 to 15 seconds will allow your heart to slow down, perhaps enough to drop out of the training zone. Personally, I find that counting my pulse for 6 seconds and multiplying the result by 10 is the easiest way to keep track of my exercising intensity.

One important note before we move on to the next chapter—all of the heart rates I have referred to in this chapter are one-minute heart rates—i.e., the number of beats your heart makes in one minute.

Well-Fit Tips

> *Rational exercise is best.*
> *Exercise with your heart rate in the training zone.*

16

Well-Fit Program

Now we come to the heart of the matter—putting it all together. In this chapter, and in the three to follow, you'll find out how to put together your own Well-Fit Program.

The program is based on a 12-week improvement period. During that time you'll lose up to 20 pounds or more, and you'll become more fit, not to mention less stressed. It takes time to change. You also need a commitment to yourself to change some things in your life—things like no exercise, over-eating—things that are hurting you. Remember, the usual recreational activities of many Americans are eating, drinking, and smoking, all done while sitting. A Well-Fit life is different. It makes and *keeps you healthy*.

FITNESS TRIAD

The Well-Fit Program has three parts. I often say that they are the three legs of a fitness stool. As you know, if one leg of a three-legged stool is shorter than the others, the stool is tilted and difficult to sit on. Remove one leg completely, and the stool is useless. So all three legs of a stool are equally important. The same applies to the parts of the Well-Fit Fitness Triad—all three are necessary, and all three are equally important. They are:

Reasonable Rest (sleep, relaxation, stress management)
Rational Exercise (aerobics, flexibility, strength)
Regulated Weight (good diet, obtaining and staying at ideal weight)

WELL-FIT PROGRAM

During the next 12 weeks you'll add all three things of the Well-Fit Triad to your life. It'll be a time of change, improvement, self-satisfaction, and fun. You'll do it in the following way.

Each day you'll eat the number of calories that'll give you a weight loss of 2 pounds per week. Also, you'll use some behavioral modification techniques to help add good eating habits to your life. You'll learn how many calories to eat and what modifications to use in Chapter 18.

Each day you'll give yourself 30 minutes to devote entirely to yourself, and those 30 minutes will be spent in stress management or exercising. At the beginning of the 12 weeks you'll have more stress management times than exercises, but by the end of the period, stress management and exercise days will alternate. You'll learn about stress management in Chapter 17, while you'll find out about exercise in Chapter 19.

This is not a rigid program. Rather, it's meant to be one that fits into your life. As a matter of fact, it's not really a "program" at all. It's a period of time during which you can teach yourself some new, productive lifestyles, hopefully adding them permanently to your life. With dedication to yourself, you'll see change and improvement—you'll get positive feedback or rewards, and these will help you continue with the program.

POSITIVE FEEDBACK

Look back to the end of Chapter 4 where you recorded your height, weight, waist, etc. Take those measurements weekly, and record them in a Well-Fit Log Book. Any small notebook can serve as a log. I suggest that you take these measurements every Friday morning, right after you get up and urinate. Why? Because we often slip on the weekends, and by taking the measurements at the end of the week before the weekend, you'll give yourself time to get back on track. Remember, positive change is important. Do everything and anything that'll help you see the positive changes in yourself. Be creative.

You might try Well-Fit Points to help keep track of your progress.

You'll add the Regulated Weight part of the Triad to your life every day, and you'll add either Reasonable Rest or Rational Exercise to your life every day also. Give yourself a Well-Fit Point each day you successfully adhere to your Regulated Weight program, and give yourself another Well-Fit Point each day you exercise or use stress management. The minimum is 2 Well-Fit Points a day, or 14 Well-Fit Points every week. Record the Points in your log like this:

R for 1 Reasonable *R*est Well-Fit Point
E for 1 Rational *E*xercise Well-Fit Point
W for 1 Regulated *W*eight Well-Fit Point

Thus each day you should have an RW or EW recorded in your log. That way you'll be able to really see how you're doing with your program. Such visual feedback will help you while you're establishing new and better habits. Eventually those new habits will become automatic parts of your life, and you'll be able to stop being so compulsive. But for now, *be compulsive.*

FINDING TIME

Many of you are probably thinking that you don't have enough time to do the things I just mentioned. That's an old, old excuse. If you're like many people, you probably are fairly disorganized, so adding some time management to your life can help find that extra 30 minutes for you. You have to establish priorities in all time management techniques. I can think of no greater priority than staying healthy, so adding these things to your life should be at the top of your list. See the resources books listed below for time management techniques.

Well-Fit Tips

> *An investment of 12 weeks can change your life.*
> *The Well-Fit Triad is:*
>   *Reasonable Rest*
>   *Rational Exercise*
>   *Regulated Weight.*
> *Give yourself 2 Well-Fit Points every day of your life.*

Resources

Bliss, E. C. *Getting Things Done.* New York, Bantam Books, 1976.

Scott, D. *How To Put More Time In Your Life.* New York, Signet Books, 1980.

Lakein, A. *How To Get Control Of Your Time And Your Life.* New York, Signet Books, 1973.

17

Well-Fit Way—Reasonable Rest

Of the three parts of the Well-Fit Triad, this is the most ignored, and it is probably the most important. As I described in Chapters 8 and 9, excessive stress can be harmful. The thing to do to be Well-Fit is to add stress management to your daily routine.

Remember, a time-out from routine is most helpful. You'll recall from the last chapter that you need to add 30 minutes of self-devotion to your day, using that time for either stress management or exercise. In Chapter 9 you learned that exercise is a tremendous stress management technique, so, in actuality, having that 30 minutes added to every one of your days gives you a daily dose of stress management even if you exercise. You earn your R Well-Fit Point.

Put that 30 minutes at the top of your list of priorities, and stick to it. I really want to drive this point home—don't neglect Reasonable Rest. You need stress management.

SLEEP

Sleep is something that everybody needs. Some people sleep more than others, some less—Benjamin Franklin, Napoleon, Thomas Edison and others got by with just a few hours of sleep each night. Whatever your sleep need, try to satisfy it every night. Develop a routine and go to bed at about the same time each night. Don't eat heavily (if at all) just before you go to bed, and don't exercise actively before retiring. These can keep you awake.

If you must eat something at bedtime, I suggest a cup of skim milk. Warm or cold, it's up to you. Some people now feel that the amino acid, tryptophan, contained within the milk can help you drift off to sleep — sort of a "natural" sleep aid. Also, you might want to do a gentle stretching program (more on stretching in Chapter 19) followed by a session of the Relaxation Response (Chapter 9) before you go to bed.

Above all, don't neglect your sleep. While you sleep your body repairs itself. Skipping sleep will reduce your stress management effectiveness. Sleep well.

REASONABLE REST WELL-FIT POINT

Now we'll sum up the things you should do to get your Reasonable Rest Well-Fit Point.

Get into the habit of getting your usual amount of sleep each night. You need it.

Reserve 30 minutes each day for yourself. On the days that you don't exercise during that time, use some sort of stress management technique. I suggest that you spend 20 minutes using the Relaxation Response. Other time-outs during the day will also help you handle stress, so try to add a few more of them, but don't neglect your basic 30 minutes.

Have fun. Don't get tied up into a dull, regimented routine. Life can be a lot of fun, and enjoying yourself is the best way to handle stress.

One final thing. Many people eat, even over-eat, while under stress. Using stress management can break you of that habit, and you'll go a long way toward earning your W Well-Fit Point as described in the next chapter.

Well-Fit Tips

Earn your R Well-Fit Point every other day.
Get regular sleep — don't neglect it.

Resources

See the Resources of Chapter 9.

18

Well-Fit Way—Regulated Weight

There are a number of medical experts who now feel that our nation's biggest health problem is bigness—obesity. When you consider that almost half of adult Americans are overweight or are obese, you can see the real magnitude of the problem.

As I said in Chapter 16, during the 12 weeks of your Well-Fit Program you can lose 20 pounds or more. That's true, and here's how you do it.

Remember back to Chapter 4 where you recorded your present weight. Get that figure and write it down on the Present Weight line below:

Present Weight_____ × 15 cal/day/pound
= _____Present calories/day

As you can see, multiply your present weight by 15, and you get an estimate of the number of calories you eat these days to maintain your present weight.

Next, write down your Present Calories/day on the top line of the formula below:

Present Calories/day _____
−1000
Reducing Calories/day_____

Subtract 1000 from Present Calories/day, and you'll have your target Reducing Calories/day. Since a pound of fat equals about 3500 calories, you can see that dropping the amount of calories you eat by 1000 each day will give you a 2-pound weight loss per week (7 × 1000 = 7000, 7000 divided by 3500 equals 2 pounds).

One note of caution. Some of you probably eat around 2000 calories or less a day. If you fit into that category, don't drop below 1200 calories/day for men or 1000 calories/day for women when you calculate your Reducing Calories/day. If you do, you'll be on a starvation diet, and you can have some problems that you'll learn about next.

SET POINT

Why not lose more than 2 pounds a week? Good question. It seems that your body will end up fighting you if you try to lose too much, too soon. It's now thought that everyone's body has an individual "set point" for weight. In other words, your body gets used to a particular weight, amount of food eaten, and level of exercise. As the commercial said, "It's not nice to fool Mother Nature"—when you diet drastically your body gets mad. To compensate for the very few calories you're giving it, your body will drop its level of metabolic activity or energy output so that it won't need the usual number of calories. It fights you.

To avoid that fight you need to lose weight gradually, and you need to find ways to lower your weight set point. Exercise, particularly aerobic exercise, will help lower your body's set point. Exercise will lower that weight set point because working out regularly increases your metabolic rate and burns off more calories. A person who exercises regularly burns off more calories at rest than does a sedentary person.

LOSING AND MAINTAINING

Now that you know your Reducing Calories/day, you can eat that amount of Calories each day, and you'll lose weight at a rational rate. Remember, during the initial part of a "diet," you lose weight rapidly, particularly on those starvation diets. That quick weight loss comes from losing *water*. But using the 1000-less-calories-a-day technique will give you a slow but steady loss of fat.

When you reach your Ideal Body Weight (see Chapter 13), you'll want to eat the number of calories you need to maintain weight. Once

WELL-FIT WAY—REGULATED WEIGHT

again, use the 15 Calories/day/pound figure as in the above formula in order to give yourself your ballpark caloric need. Weigh yourself every week, and adjust the amount that you eat as needed. Maintain your Ideal Body Weight. Keep in mind the changes that occur as time passes. With age your body's metabolic rate slowly goes down (you need 10% less calories for every 10 years after the age of 20), so keep track of your weight.

COUNTING CALORIES

Obviously, one way to keep track of what you eat is counting calories. It's really not difficult. If you buy one of the many calorie books on the market and use it for a while, you'll get to the point where you'll know the number of calories for most of the foods you eat. Think about it. You probably have a usual menu of foods, so you can easily learn the calories for your regular meals.

Buy a small food scale. That way you'll be able to measure your food portions as you prepare your foods. By the way, don't sample your food as you're cooking it! That's a subtle way to get many too many calories without realizing it.

You might want to record your calories in your Well-Fit log book. Personally, I have a small daily schedule book in my wallet, and I record my daily calories there. You might try it. You now know what your Reducing Calorie amount is, so for each meal write down the number of calories and subtract that amount from your daily allotment. Record it like this:

Breakfast – 500/1500   (Daily Calories – 2000)

The first figure is the number of calories from breakfast, the second figure is the number of calories out of the daily allotment still available. By using this method you can easily see what you've eaten, and what you still have available to eat. This way you can better plan your meals.

EXCHANGE LISTS

As you recall from Chapter 11, we all need to change our eating habits to a combination of 55% Carbohydrates, 30% Fats, and 15% Protein. Many people don't want to measure out the proper Carbohydrate/Fat/Protein levels of their food, just as many people don't want to count calories. Well, if you're in that category, I've just the thing for you—the exchange list system.

When you use the exchange list system, you don't have to count calories. That's already done for you. Instead, you select the number of calories you want to eat each day (using your Reducing Calories/day figure), and you use the exchange list's tables for that amount.

An exchange list book will give you a choice of amounts of daily calories, usually 1000, 1200, 1500, 1800, 2000, 2500, and 3000. The book gives you meat, fat, bread, vegetable, and fruit exchange lists. Suppose you choose 1800 calories. For breakfast you could have 2 fruit exchanges, 2 bread exchanges, 1 meat exchange, 1 fat exchange, and 1 cup of skim milk. You'd turn to each exchange list and find the many choices available to you in each category—for example, 1 small apple or ½ small banana, etc. See how easy it is? What's more, the exchange lists are based upon the proper combinations of Carbohydrate/Fat/Protein percentages. See the Resources List for a couple of versions of exchange lists.

BEHAVIOR MODIFICATION

Believe it or not, many of us don't know how to eat correctly. We eat out of boredom, stress, anxiety, habit, and more. We respond to external cues, like TV, walking in the front door after work, and others. We need to change in order to eat correctly, and behavior modification can help. Such techniques help you substitute good habits for bad ones. One of the most important techniques is the Eating Log. You write down everything that you eat in a log, *everything,* and you also include the place you're eating, time of day, your emotions, and other bits of information. Keeping such a log for a week or so can teach you a great deal about yourself and when and why you eat.

Of the many behavior modification techniques available, I've found the following most useful to me.

- Food Diary—By keeping a Food Diary you can learn your cues for eating.
- Cue Avoidance—Many of us eat on cue. By knowing those cues and avoiding them, you can reduce the amount of food you eat.
- Eating Room—It is often very helpful to make it a policy to eat only in one room, thus avoiding snacking elsewhere.
- Meal Beginning and End—Get in the habit of having definite beginnings and endings for your meals. Avoid that constant snacking—the calories add up. (I find that brushing my teeth after a meal is a good ending.)

- No Night Snacking – If you make it a policy to not eat for at least 2 hours before you go to bed, you'll avoid many calories.
- Long Meals – Develop the habit of having long meals. Give your body time to register the fact that you've eaten (about 20 minutes). Put your fork down between bites instead of just shoveling it in.
- Group Support – Sometimes joining a weight control group will give you the incentive to lose weight.

There are many more techniques to use, so many that I couldn't begin to list them all. I suggest that you read the books on behavior modification listed in this Chapter's Resource List.

REGULATED WEIGHT WELL-FIT POINT

Above all, earn that *W* Regulated Weight Well-Fit Point. Losing weight is not easy, contrary to many "quickie" diet ads. When you reach your Ideal Body Weight, you'll know that you've accomplished something many people can't do themselves. Remember, anything that is worth something requires self-dedication. Record that *W* each day and be proud (and healthy).

Well-Fit Tips

> *Lose 2 pounds of fat a week.*
> *Maintain your Ideal Body Weight once you reach it.*
> *Consider using Exchange Lists.*
> *Behavior Modification helps.*

Resources

> Exchange Lists:
>
> *Diet Planner.* Published by the Eli Lilly Company of Indianapolis, IN.
> Your doctor can get you a free copy of this small, very handy book.
>
> *Better Homes and Gardens Eat & Stay Slim.* Des Moines, Meredith Corp. 1979.
> This book gives the exchange list values of a number of brand name foods. You can get it in your grocery store.

Behavior Modification:

Redd, W. H., Sleator, W. *Take Charge. A Personal Guide to Behavior Modification.* New York, Random House, 1976.

Ferguson, J. M. *Learning to Eat. Behavior Modification for Weight Control.* Palo Alto, Bull Publishing Co., 1975.

19

Well-Fit Way—Rational Exercise

Did you know that 2 + 2 = 5 can be true? No, not in mathematics, of course, but in your health. There is a principle known as *synergism*, defined as "the joint action of agents so that their combined effect is greater than the algebraic sum of their individual effects." Don't get hung up on that definition from a medical dictionary, since the concept is simple; we'll use diet and exercise as examples.

Studies on many people have shown that someone who loses a lot of weight through diet alone has an almost 90% probability of gaining it all right back. That's not good odds. On the other hand, losing weight through exercise alone is a long and very slow process. Now let's look at the bright side, the synergistic side.

When you combine diet and exercise, you get a greater whole than the two parts used separately. That's right. Diet and exercise together give you the fastest and most successful way to lose weight (and become fit at the same time). That's synergism. Another way to remember it is by using the 3/10 Principle.

3/10 PRINCIPLE

The numbers 3/10 are shorthand for 300/1000. The first, 300, stands for 300 calories of exercise, while the second number, 1000, stands for 1000 calories less each day. To me, 3/10 is an easy way to remember the numbers. And why are they important?

Some fitness experts now feel that the minimum number of calories that you need to work off at one workout in order to best stimulate your body to use stored fat is 300. From the point of view of fitness, a 300-calorie workout is a very good one, especially when you keep your heart rate in the training zone (remember back to Chapter 15).

You already know about eating 1000 calories less each day in order to lose 2 pounds of fat a week (in the previous chapter). When you eat less calories in that manner in combination with a 300-calorie workout at least every other day, you give yourself the best stimulus to lose that excess weight and gain fitness. Synergism at work. Remember the 3/10 Principle. It'll help you keep in mind the proper way to stay Well-Fit.

AEROBIC EXERCISE

When you think of aerobic exercise, you have to keep a number of things in mind—intensity, frequency, duration, and modality.

The *intensity* of your exercise is how hard you are working. As you recall from Chapter 15, you can keep track of your intensity by using the exercise training-zone method. Don't get hung up on taking your pulse all of the time. Just do it about 5 minutes or so after you get started, midway through your workout, and at the end of your exercise period. Remember that there are certain things that can increase your heart rate even though you do not increase your speed—things like going up a hill, fighting a strong headwind, etc. When you encounter such conditions, adjust your speed and stay in your training zone.

How often during the week is your exercise *frequency?* Ideally, I feel that you should be working in that training-zone every other day, or 3 to 4 times a week. Obviously, you should work up to that frequency level slowly, following the schedule listed at the end of this section. If you wish to work out more frequently, you must keep in mind that your body needs time to recover from an exercise period. Exercising every day can be too much for some people, and they can become overtrained or injured. If you are one of those people who wants to work out every day, give yourself some light, easy days or one complete day off each week. We'll explore over-training in more detail in Chapter 21.

Duration is the length of each of your exercise periods. At least 20 minutes of aerobic exercise is ideal. You need that length of time with your pulse in the training-zone in order to give yourself a good exercise stimulus. Thirty minutes of exercise is probably the best, because you can do some warm-up stretching activities at the beginning of your workout and some warm-down stretching activities again at the end, giving yourself a solid 20 minutes of continuous aerobic work in the middle. Once again, you need to work up slowly to a full 30 minutes of activity using the schedule presented below. More on stretching later.

Modality is the actual exercise you choose to use during your workout. You can do anything that gets your heart rate up and keeps it up in the training-zone for the whole exercise period. Please note that your heart rate has to stay in the training-zone for the entire time. If you are using an exercise in which you stop frequently, you aren't exercising aerobically. True aerobic exercises are:

Walking   Jogging   Swimming   Bicycling

Obviously, there are many more, including dancing, jumping rope, rowing, cross-country skiing, etc. I've just listed the four above because I believe they are the most important. Let's examine each in turn.

Walking is number one. You already know how to walk; your body is used to the exercise, so you can do it fairly efficiently. If you have not exercised for a long time, walking is the modality you should start with. Believe me, a brisk walk can be a tremendous workout. Most experts will tell you that you shouldn't jump right into jogging. You need to give yourself a week or two of just walking, then add short jogging periods occasionally as you walk. Some of you may just wish to stick with walking alone.

Those of you who want to get into jogging should keep in mind the need for moderation. You body needs time to get used to any exercise, and jogging is no exception. Remember, as you jog you push yourself completely into the air with each stride, and your body has to get used to the increased impact of the exercise. Running shoes can help a great deal. Invest in a good pair, and keep them in good repair.

Swimming is a fantastic exercise. Unfortunately, many people don't know how to swim, and there aren't a whole lot of people who own pools. If you do swim, you may want to invest in a pair of swimming goggles in order to protect your eyes from the chlorine. That way you'll be able to open your eyes under water, and if you are fortunate to have the use of a pool that has lines painted on the bottom, you can periodically check your position in the water as you swim. You can swim a straight line. By the way, people with arthritis can definitely benefit from this exercise.

I'm biased. I admit it. I feel that bicycling is the best form of aerobic exercise. You're not limited to nice days—you can ride an exercise bike indoors. Your chances for injury are less than with jogging because you don't have the constant pounding of running. Of course, you do have to avoid crashing or being hit by a car, but using quiet roads or bicycle paths can help. I suggest that you wear one of the many bicycle helmets available when you ride on the road.

You must also use a bicycle that fits you. Stand over the bicycle with the horizontal bar between your legs. You should have 1 to 3 inches of clearance between that bar and your crotch. If you're resting on the bar, the bicycle is too big.

After you have found a bicycle that's the proper size, you need to adjust the saddle height. Sit on the saddle, and put the heels of your riding shoes on the pedals. Let one pedal go all the way down toward the ground. The leg on that side should just hang straight, and your pelvis should not be tilted to allow you to keep the shoe on the pedal. After you adjust the saddle height to give you that necessary straight leg extension, ride with the balls of your feet over the centers of the pedals. Don't use the heels or arches of your feet. The bicycle is not designed to be efficiently used that way. When you have the saddle at the proper height, and when you use the balls of your feet on the pedals, your legs will always have some bend in them as you ride. Also, when the saddle is at that height, you will not be able to sit on it and put both of your feet on the ground. Remember, the bicycle is meant to be ridden, not just sat upon.

One final thing about the bicycle. It's such an efficient machine that you have to be careful in order to get a good workout. You can get on a bicycle, pedal it slowly around a flat area, and actually work out less than if you had walked. You must check your heart rate and keep it in the training zone. Also remember that you're not working when you're coasting. Pedal to fitness, don't coast.

Now, on to the 12-week program. As you'll see, the program is a progressive one, giving you a slow build up. While the frequency increases over the period, the exercise duration also increases.

12-Week Well-Fit Exercise Program

Week 1	2 Sessions, 15 minutes each
Week 2	2 Sessions, 15 minutes each
Week 3	3 Sessions, 15 minutes each
Week 4	3 Sessions, 20 minutes each
Week 5	4 Sessions, 20 minutes each
Week 6	4 Sessions, 20 minutes each
Week 7	4 Sessions, 25 minutes each
Week 8	4 Sessions, 25 minutes each
Week 9	4 Sessions, 25 minutes each
Week 10	4 Sessions, 30 minutes each
Week 11	4 Sessions, 30 minutes each
Week 12	4 Sessions, 30 minutes each

Remember, you need to spend some time at the beginning and end of each exercise session doing stretching and warm-up exercises. They should take about 3 to 5 minutes each, so you can see that your actual aerobic exercise activity in this program increases slowly. At the beginning you have only about 5 minutes or so of aerobics, while at the end you get your full 20 minutes. Keep your heart rate in the training zone for each session.

Next, you might like to know how long it takes to burn off 300 calories for various exercises. As you'll see, many of them take longer than 20 minutes, but that's not a problem. The 20 minutes is your minimum. You can go longer if you wish, just as long as you build up slowly. Also, everyone has a different level of fitness, and as a result different people will need different levels of intensity in order to get in the training zone. Thus the speeds given below may be too slow for one person while too fast for another.

300 Calorie Times

Walking (3½ mph)	55 minutes
Jogging (5 mph)	30 minutes
Swimming	50 minutes
Bicycling (5 mph)	60 minutes
Bicycling (15 mph)	25 minutes

The figures given above are just guidelines. They should be raised for someone who weighs more than 155 pounds, or lowered for someone who weighs less than 155 pounds.

STRENGTH TRAINING

Every exercise program needs strength training. The quickest way to lose weight and to increase lean body mass while reducing fat body mass is to combine aerobic exercise with strength training and diet. Synergism again.

You increase your strength by giving your muscles slowly increasing loads to work against. If you have not been exercising in any way for some time, just starting the aerobic program will strengthen some of your muscles. After you've been doing the aerobic training and flexibility training for perhaps 4 to 6 weeks, you can add strength training.

You need to work your muscles against resistance, progressively increasing that resistance as you get stronger. To do that, you can use weights that you buy, or you can use things found around the house. Your kitchen has a lot of items that you can use—soup cans, pots filled with water, etc. Use your imagination!

Your strength training exercise should focus on three areas — lower body, trunk, and upper body.

The *lower body* can be strengthened several ways. You can do half-squats. Put your hands on your hips, and squat down halfway so that your thighs are just about level with the ground, then straighten back up. Do a number of those, perhaps 15 to begin, and increase the number as time passes. After the squats, do some toe raises. Just raise up on your toes, and come back down. Again, start with about 15 and work up. Finally, work on the back of your upper legs. Stand up straight and steady yourself by holding onto something. Raise one lower leg off of the floor, bringing your foot up behind you, then put the leg back down. Do that about 15 times for each leg as before, and work up. After a period of time doing those exercises, you may want to add weights, holding them in your hands or putting them on your shoulders for the squats and toe raises, and using a leg curl machine in a gym for the back of your legs.

One note of caution concerning lower body work for you who have knee problems. Many of you might have noticed that one or both of your knees snaps or crunches as you go up and down stairs, etc. If you have that problem, you need to be very careful when you weight lift. Don't do full squats, just half-squats. If you go to a gym and intend to use the leg extension machine, don't do full extensions. Bring your legs up to where they are about 30 degrees from being fully straight, and then work from there. Fully straighten your legs against resistance,

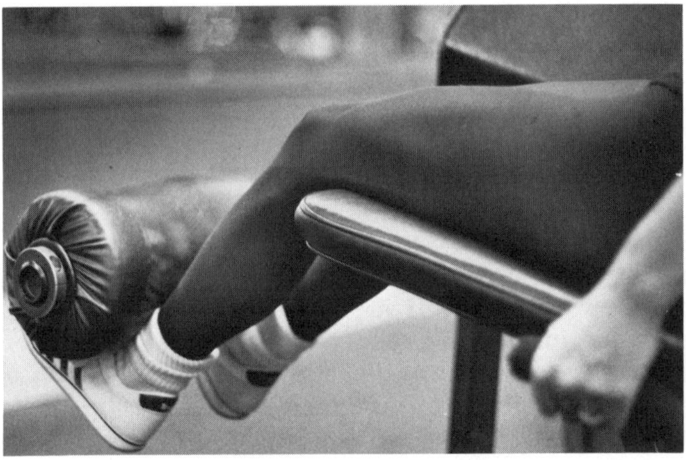

Fig. 19:1. Leg Extension Machine. This is the starting position for leg extensions. As you can see, you should start with your legs bent down only 30 degrees from horizontal. From here you must straighten your legs out completely.

WELL-FIT WAY—RATIONAL EXERCISE 75

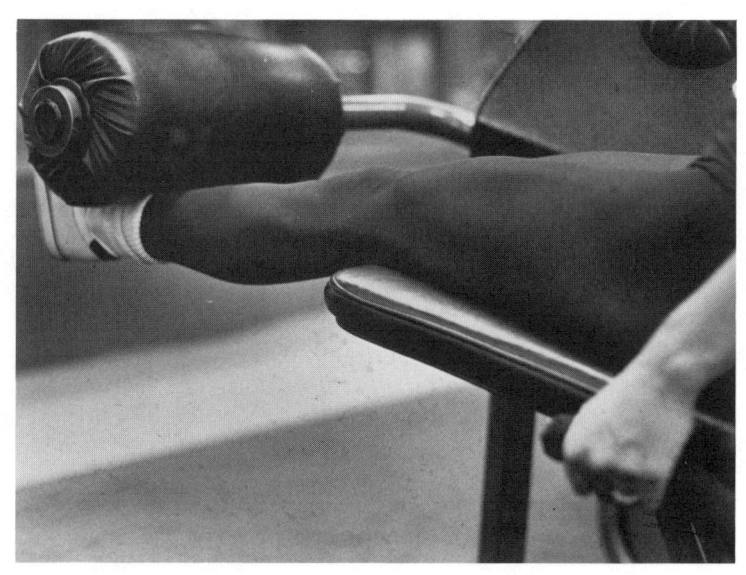

Fig. 19:2. Leg Extension Machine. This is the finishing position of the leg extension exercise. Before you let your legs go back down to 30 degrees, pause here and hold your thigh muscles in full tension for a count of 10. Then let your legs go down to the position shown in Figure 1, and do it again.

then bend them down only 30 degrees, then straighten them back out. See Figures 1 and 2 if you have any questions. Staying within 30 degrees will save your knee caps.

Now to the *trunk*. Situps will strengthen your upper abdominal muscles. To do them, lie down on the floor on your back, bend your knees and hook your toes beneath something to hold them. Put your

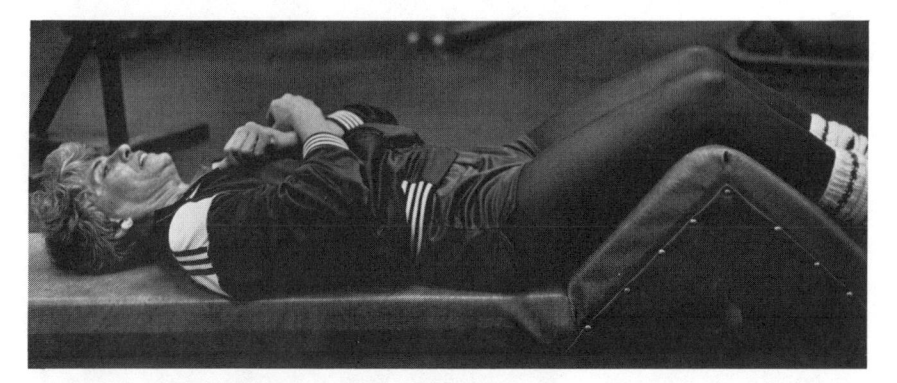

Fig. 19:3. Situps. This is the starting position for situps. As you can see, the knees are bent. If you don't have a situp board like this one, just tuck your toes under something and bend your knees.

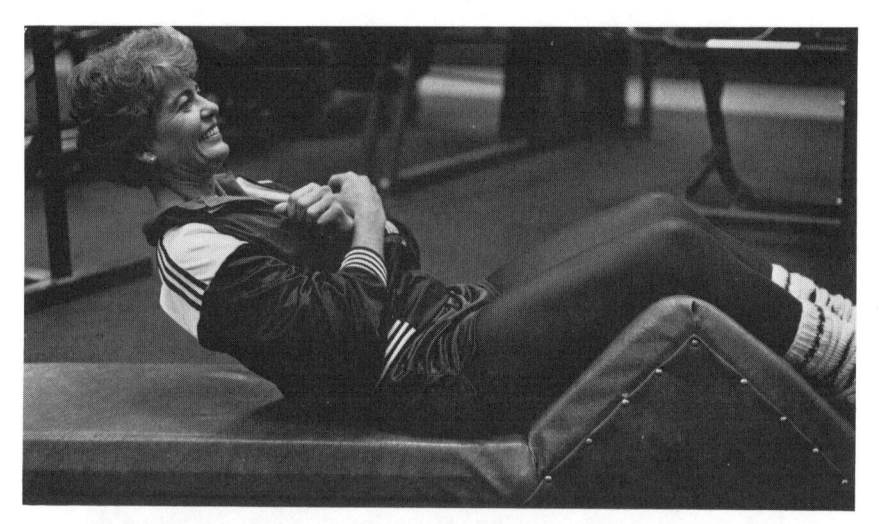

Fig. 19:4. Situps. This is the finishing position for your situp. Remember, you don't need to go all of the way up to your knees. You can put your arms on your chest like this, or you can put them behind your head or even at your sides. It's your choice.

hands on your chest, and raise your upper body up to about 30 degrees from the floor. You don't need to go all of the way up to your knees. Then lower your upper body back down to the floor. That's it, one situp, and a situp that will protect your lower back. See Figure 3 and 4.

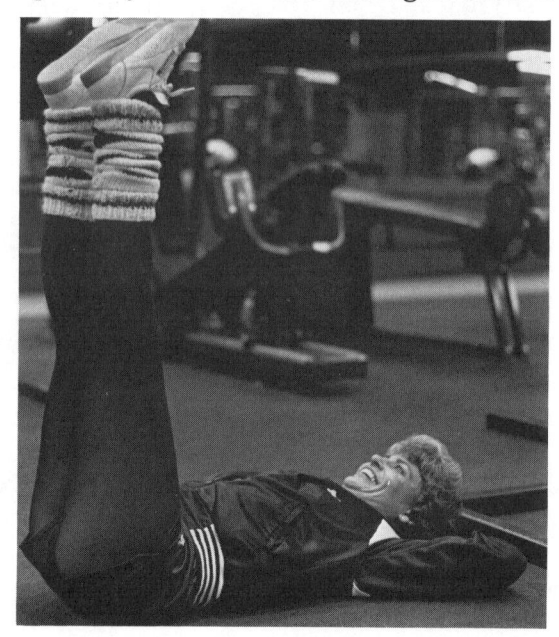

Fig. 19:5. Leg lowers. You'll begin your leg lowers from this position. If you can't keep your legs straight like this, go ahead and bend your knees a little.

WELL-FIT WAY—RATIONAL EXERCISE 77

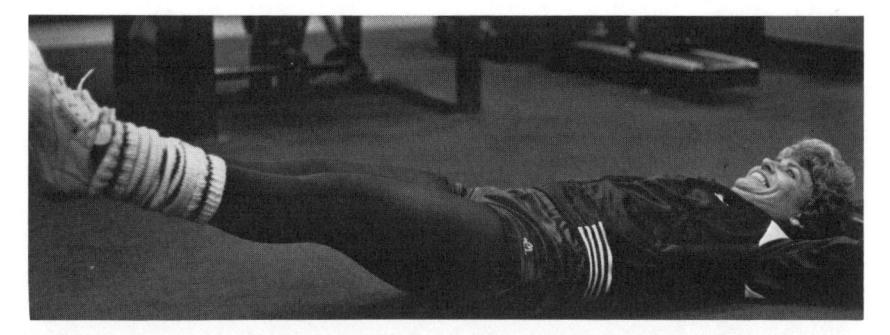

Fig. 19:6. Leg lowers. Remember, as you lower your legs, straighten them out if you had your knees bent. Stop when the small of your back begins to arch off the floor. As you raise your legs back up, you might want to bend your knees again. It'll help your back.

A beginning number of around 10 would be a good start. Increase the number gradually.

Next, leg lowers. That's right, leg lowers, not raises. Lie down on the floor on your back with your hands behind your head. Bring your legs up to vertical, pointing them toward the ceiling. You can have your knees slightly bent. Now lower your legs toward the floor slowly (straightening them at the knees if you had your knees bent), and stop when you feel that the small of your back is beginning to arch off of the floor. At that point, raise your legs back up to vertical, bending your knees as you raise them if you need to do so. See Figures 5 and 6 if you have any questions. Start out with about 5 and work up.

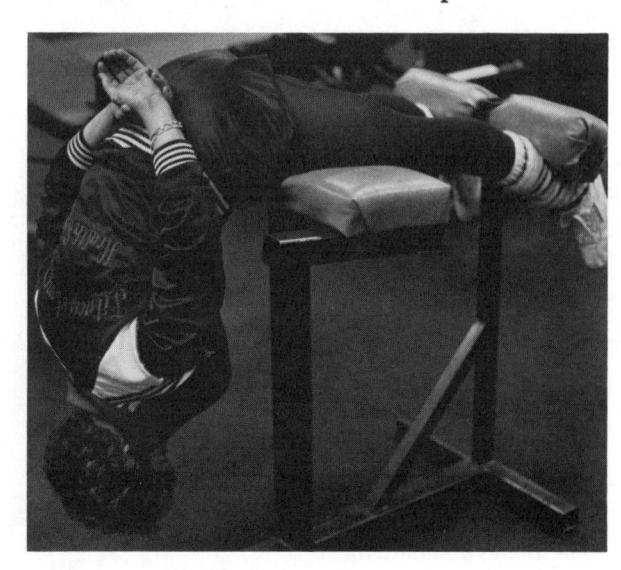

Fig. 19:7. Hyperextension. This is the starting position. Putting your hands on the small of your back like this will make the exercise a little easier.

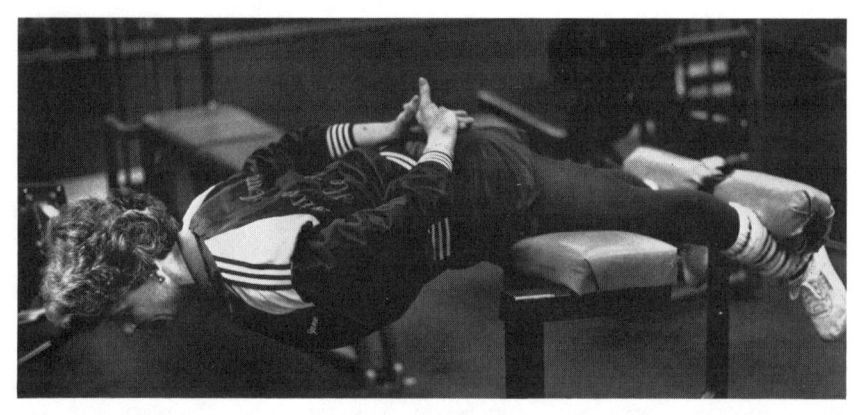

Fig. 19:8. Hyperextension. Here's where you'll finish the movement. Move slowly and steadily. Don't overdo this, and don't do it at all if your back is actively bothering you.

Your back is part of your trunk. Keep in mind that low back pain affects up to 80% of adult Americans at one time or another, so everyone needs to have a strong back. One form of back exercise is the hyperextension. Don't do this if your back is actively bothering you. You might need to go to a gym to do this, or you can have someone hold your legs at home. As you can see from Figures 7 and 8, you get on a table or something similar and bend down at the waist. You raise your upper body up until it's horizontal, and then lower it back down. This is a difficult exercise. You might want to begin with just 2 or 3 of them and work up slowly.

Twists will also help your trunk. Get a broomstick and put it behind your neck, resting on your shoulders. Put your arms out along the

Fig. 19:9. Upper body work —flyes. This is the finishing position. Start with your arms straight up in the air. Remember to bend your elbows like this as you do the exercise. Breathe in as you lower your arms, out as you raise them.

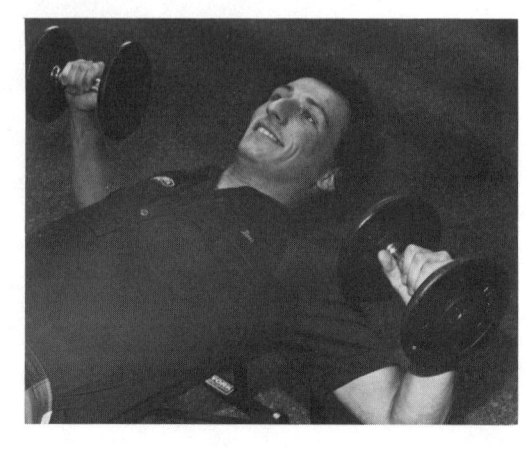

WELL-FIT WAY—RATIONAL EXERCISE 79

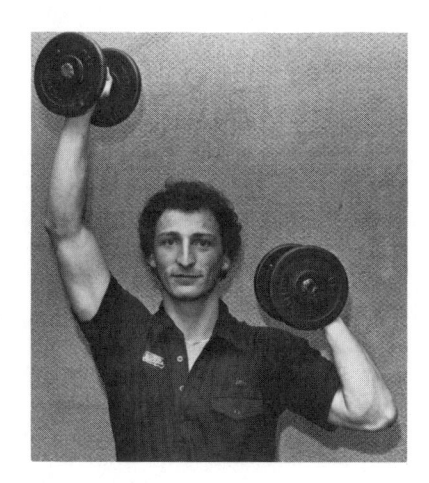

Fig. 19:10. Upper body work—presses. Here you can see both the starting and finishing positions for this exercise. You can do this by alternating your arms like this, or you can raise and lower them at the same time.

stick until they are stretched out. Twist your body around from one side to another, going as far as you can, but don't force it. Start with about 10 twists in each direction.

Finally, *upper body* work. This is something that most women need very much. For a variety of reasons, women in this society are very upper body-weak (but then again, so are a lot of men).

In Figures 9 through 12 you can see some basic upper body exercises. You don't have to go out and buy some weights for this unless you want to. Articles like soup cans, etc., will do. Start with 5 to 7 repetitions for each exercise, and then, once again, work up in both weight and repetition, reaching a repetition rate of about 12 to 15.

In all of your strength training you'll be sore for the first few days—your body needs time to get used to the exercise. Such soreness is perfectly normal, but do expect it to happen.

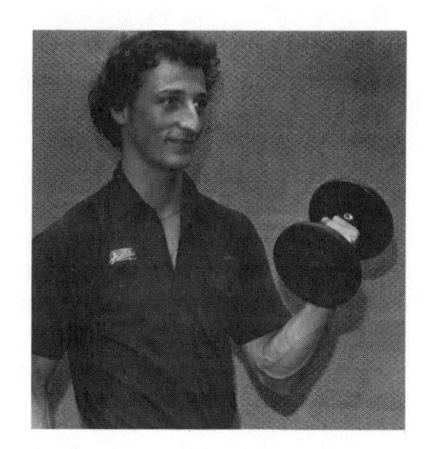

Fig. 19:11. Upper body work—curls. This exercise can be done by alternating the arms, or raising and lowering them together.

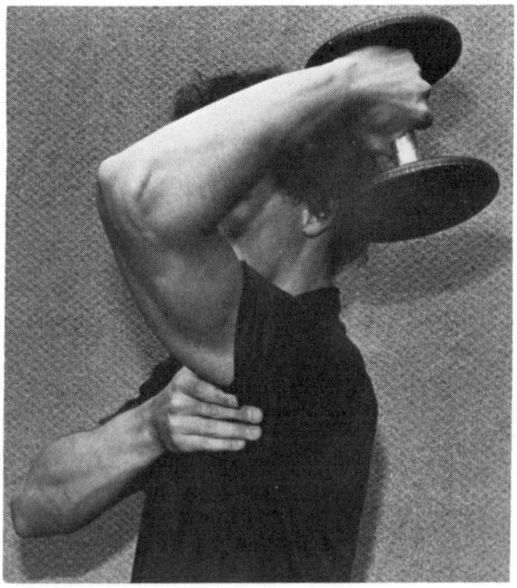

Fig. 19:12. Upper body work—triceps pushup. As you can see, this exercise is usually done one arm at a time, using the other arm to stabilize the working one. Start with your arm positioned straight up, and lower it as shown here.

STRETCHING

As your muscles strengthen they slowly get a little shorter. Because of this fact, it's very important to stretch or give yourself some flexibility training.

You must not bounce when you stretch. Instead, you slowly move until you feel a little strain on the muscles you're stretching, hold that position for 10 seconds, and then slowly ease back up. Slow and painless are the keys to effective stretching.

A stretching session both before and after each exercise period is ideal. On those days when you don't exercise, you should still do some stretching in order to stay flexible.

The muscles that most people need to stretch are the muscles of the back and the backs of the legs.

Knee to chest hugs are very helpful for stretching the back. As you can see in Figures 13 and 14, you can do this stretch with both knees or just one knee.

Next, you need to stretch the backs of your upper legs. I don't suggest toe touches while standing. Instead, sit down on the floor with your legs out flat, straight in front of you. If you can't get your legs down flat with them straight out, spread them apart a bit until you can flatten them. Lean forward from the waist until you just reach the limit of comfort, and grasp your legs with your hands. This is the position that you'll stretch from. To stretch, bend your arms out, pulling your trunk further down until you feel the stretch in the back of your

WELL-FIT WAY—RATIONAL EXERCISE 81

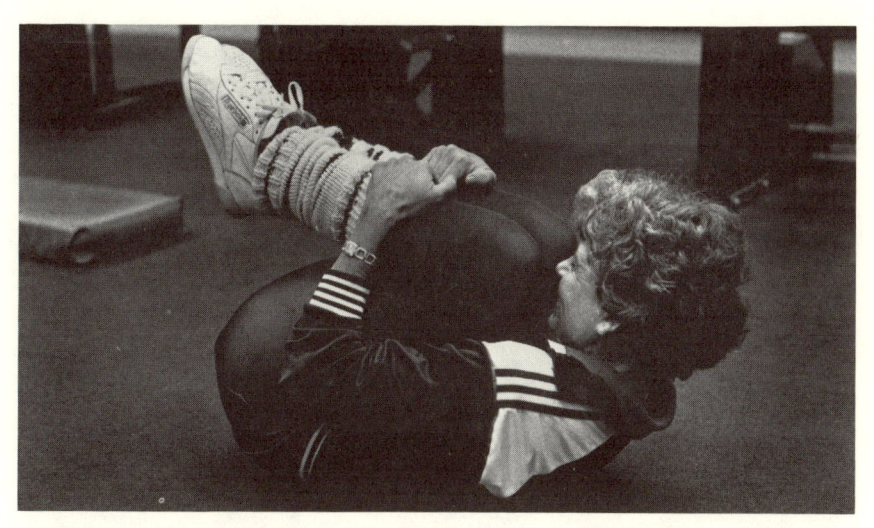

Fig. 19:13. Back stretch. This is the knee-to-chest back stretch done with both legs. When you get your knees to your chest, lift up your head as shown here.

legs, hold for 10 seconds, and slowly raise back up by straightening out your arms. Got it? If you don't, see Figures 15 and 16.

To stretch your lower leg, stand as you see in Figure 17, leaning against something. Slowly lower the heel of the foot of your back leg

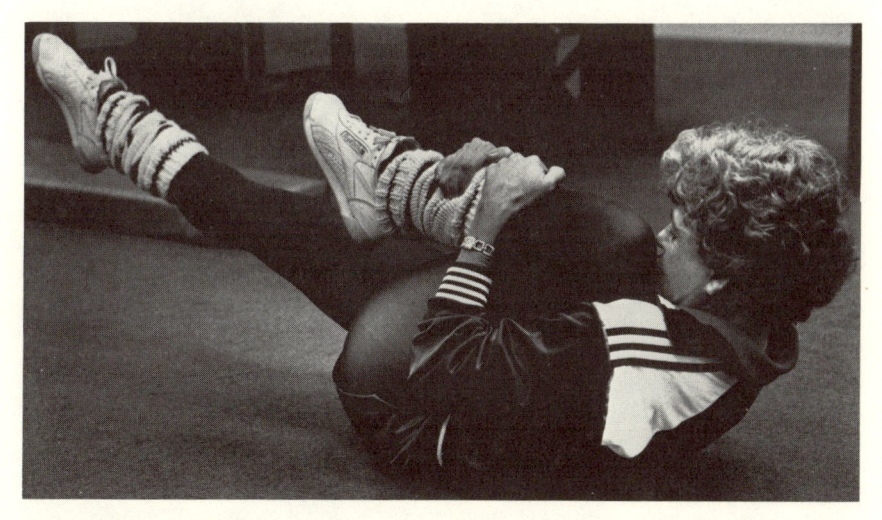

Fig. 19:14. Back stretch. Once again, the knee-to-chest back stretch, but done with only one leg. If you use this technique, alternate legs.

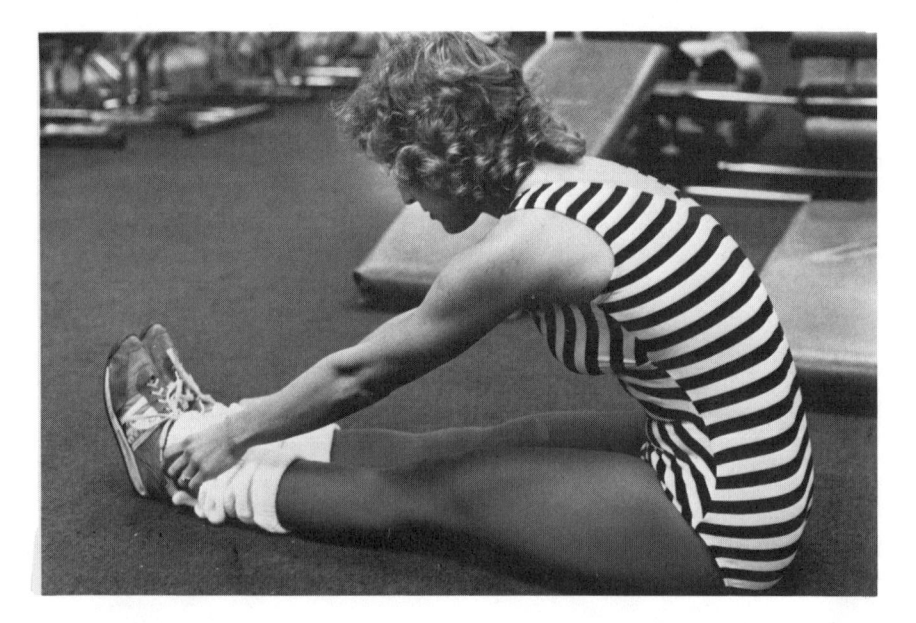

Fig. 19:15. Back of upper leg stretch. This is the starting position. Bend forward at the waist until you reach a comfortable position, then put your hands down on your legs. You may not be able to get your hands down as far as this depending on your own flexibility.

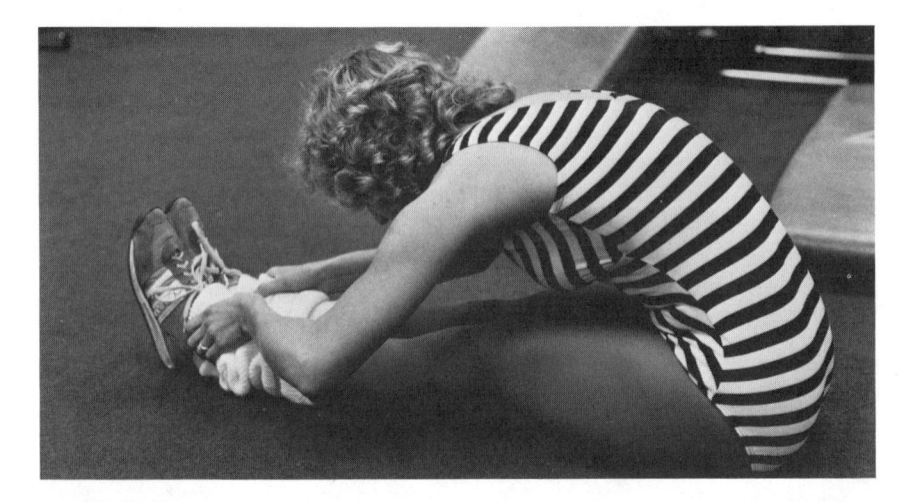

Fig. 19:16. Back of upper leg stretch. As you can see, to stretch you must push your elbows out, pulling yourself forward a bit. Pull forward until you feel the strain in the back of your legs, but not pain. Hold for 10 seconds, then release. Remember to breathe as you are stretching.

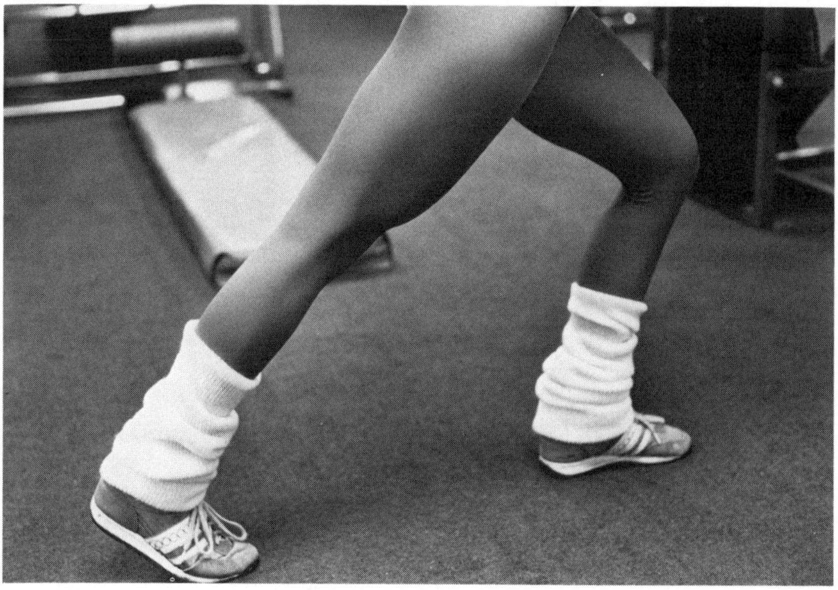

WELL-FIT WAY—RATIONAL EXERCISE

Fig. 19:17. Calf stretch. Begin the stretch in this position. Lower your heel until you feel the stretch in your calf. Don't force it to the pain threshold. Hold for 10 seconds, then raise your heel. You can do a series on one leg first and then the other, or you can alternate legs.

until you feel the stretch in your calf. Once again, hold for 10 seconds, and then slowly release.

I suggest that you do at least 5 repetitions of each stretch when you begin your flexibility training. Slowly add more repetitions as you get better. Above all, don't neglect your flexibility.

RATIONAL EXERCISE

So, there you have it—Rational Exercise. Focus on the word *Rational*. Do things in moderation. Do some stretching every day, even on the days when you don't exercise. On your exercise days, do your aerobic workout first, then your strength training. That way you'll be well warmed up.

Believe it or not, exercise is fun. When you get into it, you just might find that you actually love it. Above all, be active and get Rational Exercise the Well-Fit Way.

Well-Fit Tips

Well-Fit exercise has three parts—aerobics, strength, and flexibility.
Diet and Exercise are synergistic.
Exercise is fun.

Resources

There are countless books available on the topics of this chapter, so I've included just a few:

Darden, E. *The Superfitness Handbook*. Philadelphia, George F. Stickley Co., 1980.

Darden, E. *Your Guide to Physical Fitness*. Philadelphia, George F. Stickley Co., 1982.

Cooper, K. H. *Aerobics*. New York, Bantam Books, 1968.

Bailey, C. *Fit or Fat?* Boston, Houghton Mifflin Co., 1978.

Anderson, B. *Stretching*. Bolinas, Shelter Publications, 1980.

Krausz, J., Krausz, V. R., Harris, P. *The Bicycling Book*. New York, Dial Press, 1982.

20

Your Neighborhood Resources

When you're working on a fitness program, it is often very helpful to have some outside assistance. Obviously, any fitness program is ultimately an individual one, but help from others can ease the way. Don't neglect the various resources in your neighborhood.

HEALTH SPAS

Health spas can be tremendous sources of inspiration. Many of them offer a variety of programs, and that variety seems to be growing every day. Such a choice of things to do can help you avoid boredom with your program.

It's been said many times that a person doesn't truly value something unless he or she invests something in it. Fitness programs are no exception. The membership costs of a health spa can give you a constant reminder to use the spa—after all, you don't want to waste money!—but don't get hung up on the price. The most expensive spa might not be the best one for you.

Your health spa should be very convenient to you. Having to drive for half an hour just to get to the spa can obviously cut down on your use of the place. Another thing about convenience. Some spas are coed, while others have separate sex days. I know several women who don't like to exercise in the presence of men, and I also know other women who don't mind it. If you can't use your spa when you want to, either because of a separate sex day or inconvenient hours, your potential use of the place will also be reduced.

Check into the training of the spa personnel. You want to be able to ask questions and get help. If you find that the personnel of the place are primarily sales people with little knowledge of exercise physiology, nutrition, and so on, you might not be able to get your questions answered. As for exercise, make sure that the place has an emphasis on aerobic exercise. If the spa just stresses weight training, you won't get your money's worth.

Don't forget the local YMCA and YWCA. They often offer inexpensive programs covering a wide range of topics.

Above all, don't just leap into a health spa membership without looking into the place. You might find that your money was wasted.

WEIGHT LOSS CENTERS

Group support can be a great help during a weight loss program. Knowing that you'll be meeting each week with people who are doing the same thing that you are can really give you the incentive to lose. There are a number of well respected, national weight loss programs in this country, and many local communities also have their own organizations.

Some people would rather work on their own fitness programs alone, while others need group support. Examine yourself. If you discover that you enjoy group activities and support, you might benefit from a weight loss group. Check the Yellow Pages under "Reducing and Weight Control Services."

ORGANIZATIONS

Don't forget that organizations such as the American Heart Association, the American Cancer Society, etc., often have programs on fitness, diet, smoking cessation, and more. They are listed in the white pages of your telephone book.

FAMILY

Your family is your most important helper. It can also be your worst hindrance. It is almost impossible to make some changes in your lifestyle if your family does not support you. Let me give you an example.

Studies of how the obesity of the parents affects the weight of their children have shown that offspring of two obese parents will probably themselves be obese. Children from families in which only one parent is obese have higher chances of being overweight than those children from families in which both parents are of normal weight. In other words, your family situation has a profound influence on you and your lifestyle.

If you attempt to change your destructive lifestyles in order to achieve a Well-Fit life while the rest of your family continues along in the old ways, you'll probably never reach your goals. To counteract that problem, enlist your whole family in the change. A Well-Fit lifestyle can benefit anyone, no matter what age and sex. Be a Well-Fit Family. You'll *all* have better lives.

Well-Fit Tips

> *Choose a health spa carefully.*
> *Join an organization if necessary.*
> *Be a Well-Fit Family.*

21

Injury

The main reasons for injuries are: variation in anatomy, abrupt change in program, and over-use.

VARIATION IN ANATOMY

Unfortunately, most of us are not made perfectly. Our bodies are not absolutely symmetric. Our legs are often of different length. These anatomy problems can go undetected forever, or they can cause injuries while exercising.

The most subtle yet most dangerous anatomy variation is the unseen one of the heart. If you think back to Chapter 5, an unseen problem like this may never be an actual problem, or it can cause sudden death. Once again, if you get markedly dizzy, short of breath, or faint while exercising, get yourself checked medically before you go on with your program

A very common variation in anatomy is an increase in the Q angle. The Q angle is the angle of your leg at the knee. You've seen an increased Q angle – someone who is "knocked-kneed" has one on each leg. This can cause knee problems, mainly for runners, but it can also affect bicyclists. If you find that you are constantly having knee pain, you might want to be checked by an orthopedic surgeon.

So if you are having a chronic problem with exercise, it might be caused by a variation in your anatomy. Get yourself checked out.

INJURY

CHANGE IN PROGRAM

I have been constantly stressing the need for moderation and gradual change in order to give your body time to adapt. You can cause an injury if you ignore those points and make a dramatic change in your training program. I'm talking about suddenly increasing your miles, or abruptly increasing your speed, or dramatically changing your program. Give your body time to adapt. Do things gradually, and listen to your body as you make changes. *You are the expert on yourself.* You are the only one who can feel *your* pain.

OVER-USE

There can come a time when you ask your body to do something for too long. You can sustain an over-use injury, problems such as shin splints, or stress fractures in running. Bicyclists can develop boils, or pain on urination, or numb hands or penises. These problems can happen to anyone. To prevent them, I suggest that you stick to the every-other-day exercising routine I mentioned in Chapter 19. Give yourself rest days. In reality, your rest days are just as important to your fitness program as are your exercise days. You need that recovery time; but don't make it all of the time and never exercise!

OVER-TRAINING

One common form of over-use injury is over-training. If you follow the gradual buildup of the 12-week program, you probably won't have this problem. Those of you who ask too much of yourselves by training too hard or too long or too often might develop the signs and symptoms of over-training. They are:

Marked fatigue
Elevated resting heart rate
Elevated blood pressure
Marked weight loss
Difficulty sleeping
Irritability
Loss of sexual libido
Loss of interest in exercise

These problems can sneak up on you gradually, so it is a good idea for you to monitor yourself. Take your resting pulse fairly often. If it's more than 4 to 5 beats higher than usual, give yourself some rest. Keep track of your weight. I know that most people want to lose weight, but remember that you want to lose it gradually, and when you reach your ideal weight you want to stay there. Watch how you feel and how well you sleep. If you notice some problems with these, rest. Above all, listen to yourself!

STRAINS AND SPRAINS

A strain is an injury to muscle or tendon, the structure that attaches muscle to bone. When you hear the statement, "I pulled a muscle," that's actually a muscular strain. If you're exercising and you suddenly get a severe pain in one of your working muscles, you might have strained it. One common place for muscular strains is the back of the upper leg or the hamstring muscles.

On the other hand, a sprain is an injury to ligaments or the structures that hold bones together. Perhaps the most common sprain is the twisted or sprained ankle.

In both strains and sprains fibers of muscle, tendon, or ligament are torn. A simple strain or sprain has only microscopic damage, but damage that causes pain. More severe injuries of this sort involve partial or complete tears of these structures. In those cases more pain and swelling are experienced.

Pain and swelling – the cardinal signs of injury. If you have such an injury, remember the R.I.C.E. method of treatment. R.I.C.E. stands for:

R..rest
I..ice
C..compression
E..elevation

Rest the injured area. Put ice on it. Put the ice in an ice bag or a plastic bag and put the bag directly on the skin over the injury. It will be uncomfortable for a while, but your skin will go numb. Leave the ice there for 15 to 20 minutes, and repeat the process about 4 to 6 times a day for 2 to 3 days. Don't use any heat during that period or you'll make matters worse – you're trying to prevent swelling. Use something like an Ace wrap on the area to give some compression, again trying to prevent swelling. Finally, keep the area elevated so that gravity can help prevent swelling. After the ice period, begin to use warm soaks for 20 minutes 4 to 6 times a day. Slowly resume use of the injured area. Remember to work back up gradually.

FRACTURES

Let me clear up one thing right now – "broken" and "fractured" mean the same thing. A bone that is cracked or completely broken apart is fractured or broken. If you happen to fall or be hit, and you notice an area of deformity, swelling, and pain, you might have a fracture. If that happens, immobilize the area, put ice on it and elevate it, and see a doctor as quickly as possible.

SELF-HELP

The key to self-help is awareness of your body. Listen to it. If you feel pain, realize that your body is telling you that something is wrong. *If it hurts, don't do it!* As simple as that sounds, there are many, many people who ignore it. You have to expect some discomfort while you train. The statement "No pain, no gain" refers to training discomfort. When I say that if it hurts, don't do it, I'm talking about injury pain. You'll know the difference. Remember, taking care of yourself is the Well-Fit life.

Well-Fit Tips

> *Injuries are often caused by mistakes in training.*
> *Avoid over-training.*
> *Remember R.I.C.E.*
> *Listen to your body.*

Resources

> Mangi, R., Jokl, P., Dayton, O. W. *The Runner's Complete Medical Guide.* New York, Summit Books, 1979.
>
> Mirkin, G., Hoffman, M. *The Sportsmedicine Book.* Boston, Little, Brown and Co., 1978.
>
> Darden, E. *The Athlete's Guide to Sports Medicine.* Chicago, Contemporary Books, 1981.

22

Feminine Fitness

Many women have concerns about exercise. Many feel that exercise is not feminine—there is that old saying that men sweat and women glow. Wrong! Exercise is feminine. *Fitness* is feminine, and feminine fitness is more than just being at the ideal weight.

However, women who exercise need to know several things in order to prevent problems.

PREGNANCY

A number of doctors feel that a woman who has been following a regular exercise program before pregnancy can continue that program during pregnancy. Of course, as the abdomen gets larger she would have to alter some of her exercise routines, but she can continue doing them. On the other hand, a woman who has been inactive for some time before pregnancy should wait to start an exercise program until after she delivers the baby. The baby may have some problems if the mother is still trying to get into shape.

MENSTRUATION

Exercise can help relieve the pain of menstrual cramps. It's perfectly all right to continue to exercise while menstruating; it will not harm you.

There is one area of exercise that can affect menstruation—dropping too low in weight. When a woman loses too much weight, she can stop menstruating. This happens fairly often in those athletes who need low body weights, such as runners. When such a person backs off on her training and gains some weight, she will usually have menstrual periods again, and fertility is rarely affected.

BRAS

It is very helpful to wear a bra while exercising. Women runners can get Jogger's Nipples from the rubbing of the nipples on the shirt while running. Women with large breasts should always wear a bra while working out. There is increased comfort, and the breasts are better protected. A number of sports bras are now on the market.

MISCONCEPTIONS

The main thing women must do is overcome those misconceptions about the female and exercise. Unfortunately, there still are a number of people who want to continue to believe that exercise is not feminine. Don't believe them. Do exercise and have fun.

Well-Fit Tips

> *Exercise is feminine.*
> *A woman who has exercised regularly can continue to do so while pregnant.*
> *You can exercise while menstruating.*
> *Wear a bra while exercising.*

23

Body Parts

Let's spend a little time talking about several areas of your body that need some special care and which are overlooked quite frequently.

TEETH

Good teeth are necessary for a Well-Fit life. Now I know that you're probably sick and tired of hearing "brush your teeth three times a day," but good tooth care is essential to keeping your teeth. Unfortunately, our modern way of life seems to have a very negative effect on teeth. The amount of sugar and other refined foods that we eat does our teeth in. This has not always been true. Remains of people from several thousand years ago discovered in the area of Egypt all had all their teeth! The archeologists found that those people had other bodily problems besides tooth decay. Their diets were low in refined foods, but their teeth were sound!

Unsound teeth is the order of the day in our modern world. As a matter of fact, dental cavities are probably the most common degenerative disease on earth. It's believed that almost all Americans have some form of tooth decay, and about half of American adults wil have lost all of their teeth by the age of 55. The price we Americans pay for all of this is about $10 billion each year.

The damage to the teeth that causes these expenses results from the action of bacteria. Contained in the sticky plaque that sits on most people's teeth, mouth bacteria use the refined sugars that we eat as food for themselves. Unfortunately, as those germs do their work fermenting the sugars, organic acids are produced that eat away at the tooth enamel, decalcifying the surface. When that happens the bacteria can move into the inside of the teeth and set up shop. Given enough time, they then destroy the affected teeth. Cavities are the result.

The plaque mentioned above is a gummy substance that sticks to the teeth, and it's a perfect place for bacteria to live. Plaque needs to be removed daily. The best way to remove it is to use dental floss followed by brushing. A careful flossing once a day and brushing the teeth after each meal can really help to reduce plaque and subsequent decay.

Another tooth disease that contributes to the $10 billion expense is periodontal or gum disease. Once again, bacteria are probably the cause. Some people are more susceptible to this problem, particularly people with chronic illnesses, alcoholics, and smokers. The resistance of people to the disease varies. Oral hygiene similar to that outlined above is the best way to prevent this problem.

Above all, preventive teeth care is the best care of all. It's distressing to encounter people in their early 20's who are wearing partial or full dentures. *Take care of your teeth.*

BACK

As you recall, 80% of adult Americans have low back pain sometime during their lives. It's a tremendous problem that costs us at least $1 billion each year, yet for the most part, it is a preventable problem.

Most low back pain is caused by lack of muscular strength and poor posture. As we grow older our abdominal muscles become weaker and the amount of fat on top of those muscles grows. As the belly grows and the muscles weaken, the posture deteriorates. "Sway backs" abound. And low back pain results.

Obviously, the way to prevent this is to keep the amount of fat down, and the muscular strength up. The trunk exercises described in Chapter 19 can help a great deal, as can losing weight. Remember, it is not written in stone that we *have to* gain weight as we grow older. We do that to ourselves. Use your Well-Fit Program to lose that excess weight and increase your muscular strength. Your back will thank you!

SKIN

There are many skin problems, but given our sun worshipping habits, it would be a good idea to discuss briefly the skin problems associated with sun exposure. Most people equate a good sun tan with good health, but that's not always true.

Believe it or not, there are more than 25 diseases associated with exposure of the human skin to sunlight. They range from premature aging of the skin, cancer, photosensitivity reactions, alterations of immune system function, and more. All in all, the sun is not to be played with.

Fair-skinned people should be extremely careful in the sun. If you know that you sunburn easily, you might want to use one of the better sunscreens on the market. You really should avoid getting sunburned, because it's repeated episodes of excessive sun exposure that cause problems, especially skin cancer.

Treat your skin with care. It's the largest organ of your body, and it serves you well. Contrary to popular belief, a good sun tan is not necessarily part of a Well-Fit life.

Well-Fit Tips

> *Care for your teeth — you need them.*
> *Protect your back by staying strong and at normal weight.*
> *Avoid prolonged exposure to the sun.*

24

Fads

The areas of fitness, diet, weight control, exercise, and so on all contain many fads. Unfortunately, we Americans look for the quick, no-work way out of a situation. Fads offer the promise of quick, painless results. They can also hurt you, so it's a good idea to have some knowledge of the various fad programs being used today.

FAD DIETS

This is probably the most fad-ridden area in the health field. Lose weight overnight! Go on the candy diet and lose 20 pounds! Eat anything you want in any quantity and still lose weight! Take a pill and lose your pounds! Just look at the various magazines available in the grocery store. You'll see different diets every week. Ask yourself—if these diets really worked, why are there so many more cropping up?

Remember that a fad diet does not change your basic eating patterns. When you go off the diet you will probably return to your old ways of eating, and you'll probably return to your old weight (if not more). These diets take weight off, but for the most part they don't keep it off. We end up losing and gaining, losing and gaining, over and over again. As the Harvard nutritionist Dr. Jean Mayer says, this is "the rhythm method of girth control."

If you choose to use one of the fad diets, you should know what you're going to do to yourself. Such diets are not without problems. They generally fall into several categories as follows.

Low Carbohydrate Diets

Low carbohydrate diets are just that—low in carbohydrates. They usually are either high in protein or high in fat, or both. Whatever the type, these diets produce a quick weight loss initially because of the water loss that goes with the body's use of stored carbohydrates that are not replaced. Such water loss gives the dieter a sense of early accomplishment, but it is not a true fat loss. Also, these types of diets tend to throw the body into a state of ketosis. Ketone bodies are produced because carbohydrates are not available for energy production. Besides producing bad breath, these diets put quite a working load on the kidneys, so if the dieter has kidney disease, problems may result. Also, they can cause weakness, fatigue, and sometimes low blood pressure. Some of the diets in this category are the:

"Drinking Man's Diet"
"Stillman Diet"
"Scarsdale Diet"
"Dr. Atkins' Diet Revolution"

High Carbohydrate Diets

As the name implies, these diets are high in carbohydrates. If you are not careful, you might not get your necessary balanced protein while you follow one of these programs. Also, they have a tendency, at least at first, to cause intestinal gas and sometimes diarrhea. The diarrhea will obviously help you to lose weight, but once again it's not real fat loss. These programs are often difficult to stay on, but some of them do have the advantage of being fairly nutritionally sound. Unfortunately, others of them are not at all nutritionally valid. Consider the program well before you begin using it. A couple of diets in this category are the:

"Pritikin Program"
"Beverly Hills Diet"

Protein Sparing Fasts

During fasting, or when you don't eat anything, you lose both fat body mass and lean body mass. You lose some of your protein. In an effort to combat this fact, some modified fasts try to spare the protein, losing only fat. Unfortunately, they are not always successful, and they also have a tendency to kill people. A number of deaths have been reported connected with the use of these protein sparing liquids. Such deaths seem to be the result of heart arrhythmias (abnormal beats) or damage to the heart muscle itself. Recently a new type of diet in this category has reached the market, one that claims to have corrected the problems of the older versions that killed people, but the jury is still out on it. Fasting is a very stressful way to lose weight. If you have any major medical problems, such as heart disease, diabetes, high blood pressure, etc., you should not go on one of these diets unless you have close medical supervision. A couple of the diets included in this category are the:

"Last Chance Diet"
"Cambridge Diet"

There are other types of diets available, but the best type is that presented in Chapters 11 and 18. The only good way to lose weight and keep it off is to reduce your calories while continuing to eat properly balanced meals. Changing your eating habits for the better is also necessary. Once again, remember that it took some time to gain the excess weight, and it'll take some time to get it back off.

DIET AIDS

Also on the market are a number of diet aids. They, too, have their problems, and you need to know about them before you use the products. We'll examine a few of them.

Diet Pills

We covered these products in Chapter 7. The main ingredient in them is phenylpropanolamine. As you recall, this drug is used in many cold remedies. Its use is not without some hazard, and its effectiveness as an appetite reducer is not entirely clear. Since this product is not entirely safe, I don't recommend its use, but if you must experiment, be careful.

HCG

HCG stands for Human Chorionic Gonadotropin, a hormone found in pregnant women. Injections of this substance are supposed to suppress your appetite. Whether or not it actually does is not clear. As with many of these products, you can't eliminate the so-called "placebo" effect. A placebo is something that does absolutely nothing by itself, a "sugar pill," but its use makes the person taking it *believe* that something has helped his or her problem. The mind is a very powerful force, and if you really believe that something will help you, it often will. But don't use HCG.

Starch Blockers

For more than 25 years it's been known that certain plant foods such as wheat, kidney beans, and the like, contain a substance that stops the action of one of the digestive enzymes that work on starches. So the thought was that by using this substance, one could eat starches and not digest them, without getting the calories or gaining weight. In other words, a person could eat a lot and yet not absorb that many calories. What a good deal — too bad it doesn't work!

A number of studies on these starch blockers have shown that they do not work. One such study published in December of 1982 suggests that the reason for the lack of effectiveness of these products is that the enzyme involved is secreted by the body in such large amounts that the blocker cannot shut down all of it. Whatever the reason, these products have been removed from the market by the FDA pending further testing. Be aware that a number of them are still available. But they don't work.

SPOT REDUCING PRODUCTS

If you look in many magazines you'll see numerous ads for special creams, lotions, machines, wraps, etc., that all claim to enable you to lose fat in one area of your body. Forget it. They don't work either.

Spot reducing just does not happen. You cannot lose fat from just one place. As you lose weight, you reduce the amount of fat stored in your fat cells *all over your body*. Obviously, those areas that have the most fat will show the slowest changes, and these areas are often the ones people want most to spot reduce.

One group wanted to study spot reducing to see if it was possible to reduce the amount of fat in one spot. They did fat biopsies over their abdominal muscles, measuring the amount of fat there. Then they went on a rigorous program of abdominal exercises for a number of weeks. At the end of the training period they had rock-hard abdominal muscles, but repeat biopsies of the fat over those muscles showed no change. No spot reduction of fat occurred. Don't buy those products.

QUICKIE FITNESS

You might run across books, articles, etc., that tell you that you can become fit doing only a couple of minutes of exercise a day ... Quickie fitness. By now you know that something for nothing doesn't exist. Don't believe such claims. You must give your body regular training sessions with your heart rate in the training zone, and those sessions must be fairly frequent.

An exercise study reported in the scientific literature a couple of years ago was incorrectly reported by a popular magazine. In the study a group of people were placed on a rigorous 6-day-a-week training program for 10 weeks. They all increased their fitness. Their intensity of exercise was kept almost at maximum. At the end of the 10 weeks the group was divided into two groups, one of which went on a 4-time-a-week maintenance exercise program while the other group went on a 2-day-a-week routine. After staying on their respective programs for another 10 weeks, both groups were retested. No difference in fitness was found, so the popular magazine reported that you could maintain fitness with 2 exercise periods a week. Unfortunately, that magazine forgot to mention that both groups continued to utilize an exercise intensity near maximum, an intensity that few people can attain. That high intensity was what kept the groups equal. So, when you read some claim like that, question it. Don't take every printed conclusion at face value. If necessary, read the *original work* so that you can make up your own mind.

VITAMINS

The final fad I want to discuss is vitamins. As I write this I feel that fictional massive *Guns of Navarone* are being trained upon me by those people who emphatically believe in vitamins. Before you shoot, consider a few things.

As you recall from Chapter 11, vitamins are cofactors, or helpers in chemical reactions. Very small amounts of them are necessary in order to accomplish these tasks. As a matter of fact, Jane Brody in her *Nutrition Book* states that all of the vitamins we need each day amount to one-eighth of a teaspoon!

Unfortunately, much of the modern refining and processing that we do to our food removes vitamins, and we also don't always eat the ideal balanced diet. So some vitamin supplementation may be necessary. The problem concerning fad use of vitamins lies in taking huge doses of them, that is, using megadoses.

There is a very common attitude that holds that if a little of something is needed, a lot of it will be even better. Some megadose vitamin use has been found to act as a drug. This can help some problems, but that knowledge seems to have led the vitamin enthusiasts to conclude that they should take all vitamins in megadoses. Much of that overdose will be eliminated (it's been said that we Americans have the most vitamin-enriched sewage in the world) but some will not, especially the fat soluble vitamins. Too much vitamin A, for example, can make you sick, and far too much can actually kill you. Don't overdose on vitamins. Don't get hung-up on the word-play of vitamin – vitamin = vital – just because you feel run down. It doesn't mean that taking a vitamin will pep you up (except for the placebo effect). If you still feel you want to "make sure" that you're getting enough, just take one of the one-a-day combinations on the market.

Another common attitude concerning vitamins is that natural vitamins are better than synthetic ones. Wrong – the molecules are the same. A natural vitamin does not carry with it some mysterious "aura" of life. Both chemicals work the same way. Of course, if you feel that you must take vitamins, and if you can afford the often more expensive "natural" ones, go ahead. The placebo effect may once again help you. Just have an objective understanding about what you're doing.

Remember, a Well-Fit diet is a balanced diet, one that will give you all of the vitamins and minerals that you need without supplements.

Watch out for fads. Develop the habit of questioning outlandish claims. Be an aware consumer. Don't waste your time, money, and good health.

Well-Fit Tips

Be aware that fads are everywhere.
Be an aware consumer.

Resources

Barrett, S. (Ed.) *The Health Robbers*. Philadelphia, George F. Stickley Co., 1980.

Herbert, V., Barrett, S. *Vitamins and "Health Foods": The Great American Hustle*. Philadelphia, George F. Stickley Co., 1981.

25

Your Well-Fit Lifetime

A dedication to a Well-Fit life can increase your quality of life. That's an important fact. Even if you live a long life, if that life is spent in a state of ill health, you probably won't enjoy it. I recently saw a T-shirt that said "If I had known that I was going to live this long, I would have taken better care of myself." It's amazing to see the number of people who didn't care for themselves, and their lives don't seem to be too happy now. It's difficult to be happy, for example, when you can't walk across a room without getting short of breath. To successfully live a Well-Fit life you need to break the bonds of dependency and live as an independent person.

DEPENDENCY

We have become a society of dependent people, especially when it comes to our health care. A number of things seem to have contributed to that fact.

Ours is now a very complex society. It's difficult to understand everything, so we have to specialize. We thus depend upon others in the areas that we don't know about. At the same time, we don't want to experience failure. After all, isn't "American" the best? So, we're afraid to experiment, particularly when it comes to our health. Essentially, we have lost the ability to trust our own judgments when we're dealing with health matters.

At the same time that we've developed this dependency, we've come to believe that perfection is possible in health care. Television is one of the main reasons for this incorrect assumption. No matter what we do to ourselves, modern medicine can fix it. Would that it were so! This belief allows us to continue with our dependency (no need to question perfection), and it also gives us the opportunity to hold on to our denials.

Many of us are well aware of our use of denial as we continue to do things that harm us. If we were to overcome that denial, the possible consequences of our actions would come crashing down on us, but having that confidence in medicine allows us to deny all we want. In the long run, such dependency and self-abuse adversely affect our health.

It's time to become our own health experts. After all, it's our health, isn't it? We are the ones who suffer if it goes bad. All we need do to correct things is to acknowledge our self-responsibility, accept the need for experimentation, and live a Well-Fit life.

CHANCE

As you now know, living a Well-Fit life will help you in many ways. I'd like to say that you would not get any major medical problems, but, unfortunately, that's not so. Chance still operates. Even if you are in perfect health, something can happen to you. One nice thing is that such a problem might not affect a Well-Fit individual quite so seriously since such a person has healthy tissues.

Don't focus on the possibility of a chance medical problem. If it happens, it happens. Instead, enjoy your improved quality of life and your longer life expectancy. Just remember, your body doesn't think, *you* think, and your thinking can help your health if you do the right things. Live life the Well-Fit Way.

Well-Fit Tips

> *Be an independent Well-Fit person.*
> *Enjoy your improved quality of life and your increased life expectancy.*

Epilogue

So there you have it—the information that constitutes the first step of your "thousand mile journey." This book is your resource to use as you explore yourself and learn the things about yourself that will enable you to become Well-Fit. Use the information contained within as suggestions. Think about them. Make your own judgments. Decide how you want to live your life. It's your life to "make or break," and I hope that by using this book and the others I have recommended, you'll make a better life for yourself.

Remember, a Well-Fit life is based upon the fitness triad: Reasonable Rest, Rational Exercise, and Regulated Weight. These are the "three R's" of health. But don't become too obsessed with them, because they're simply guidelines to follow.

As a Well-Fit person you'll have more life to enjoy. What better can you give yourself? And by being Well-Fit, you can probably avoid an early visit to me in the Emergency Department. As that television commercial put it, "you can see me now, or you can see me later." I'd like to see you much, much later (if at all) as a doctor. I don't at all enjoy seeing the consequences of self-abuse. Follow the suggestions in this book, and you'll avoid self-abuse.

Once again, welcome to the Well-Fit Way. Enjoy it.

Index

Numbers in *italics* indicate figures.

Accidents, auto, incidence of, 6
   seat belts and, 6
Aerobic capacity, increase in, in long-term exercise, 53
Aerobic exercise, 52–53, 70, 73
   benefits of, 53–54
   cardiac changes in, 53
   definition of, 52–53
   duration of, 70–71
   examples of, 71–72
   frequency of, 70
   intensity of, 70
   modality of, 71
   pulmonary changes in, 53
Aerobics, Kenneth Cooper and, 17
Age, as risk factor in exercise, 19
   check-up and, 19
Alcohol, consumption of, *one*, 25–26
   stopping, 26
   in U.S., 25
   -related problems, cost of, 5, 25
   physical, 25
Alcoholics Anonymous, 26
American College of Sports Medicine, and persons at risk in exercise program, 19
Amino acids, essential, 43
Anatomy, variation in, injuries in, 88
Anger, when problem not fixed, 2
Anorexia nervosa, 49–50
Anxiety, as necessary part of life, 32
   coping with, 29
   desire to reduce, 29
Arthritis, degenerative, in obesity, 48
Atherosclerosis, in excess fat intake, 40
Auto accidents, incidence of, 6
   seat belts and, 6

Back, low, pain in, causes of, 95
   cost of, 5, 95
   obesity in, 6
   prevention of, 95
   stretching of, 80, *81*
   strong, exercise for, *77*, *78*, *78*
Bacteria, in tooth decay, 95

Basic Four Food Groups, 41–42
Beef, Kobe, 37–38
Behavior modification, in fitness program, 59
  resource reading on, 68
  in weight loss program, 66
  techniques for, 66–67
Benson, Herbert, Relaxation Response of, 34
Bicycle, efficient use of, 72
  proper size of, 72
  stationary, as test for exercise program, 19
Bicycling, as aerobic exercise, 71–72
Big Mac syndrome, and correction of problems, 2
Blood, fats in, as risk factor, 18–19
Blood pressure, high, as risk factor, 18
  as "silent killer," 18
  obesity and, 6, 47
  resting, assessment of, 15
Blood volume, in long-term exercise, 53
Body, abuse of, factors contributing to, 7
  shortening of life expectancy through, 10
  as not perfect, 2–3
  breakdown of, slowing of, 12
  helping of, to help self, 1–2
  influence over, 1
  lack of care of, in belief in modern medicine, 3
  lower, strength training for, 74, 74, 75
  measurements, height, 14
    waist circumference, 14
    weight, 14
  organs of, degeneration of, 7
  parts, special care of, 94–96
  repair of, itself, 2
  in response to stress, 29
  taking better care of, need for, 3
  understanding of, 1
  upper, strength training for, 78, 79, 79, 80
Weight, Ideal (IBW), 50–51
  maintenance of, 64–65
  well-tuned, in long-term exercise, 53
Body fat, energy stored as, 46
  functions of, 46
  and health problems, 47–49
  regular, 47
  subcutaneous layer of, 47
Body mass, fat, 47
  lean, definition of, 46–47
Body Mass Index (BMI), calculation of, 16
  definition of, 16
  explanation of assessment of, 49
Body Weight, Ideal (IBW), 50–51
  maintenance of, 64–65
Bone(s), fractured, definition of, 91
  management in, 91
Book(s), Calorie, for calorie counting, 65
  Eating Log, use of, 66
  exchange list, in weight loss program, 66, 67
  log, of stress situations, 32
  Well-Fit, recording of daily calorie intake in, 65
Bras, for exercise, 93
Breads, consumption of, 39
Breath, shortness of, simulation of, 6–7
Brody, Jane, and vitamins, 101
Bronchitis, chronic, in smoking, 22
Business, health of employees influencing, 5–6

Caesar, Julius, 36
Caffeine, as stimulant, 26

and health problems, 26
  sources of, 26
Calf, stretching of, 81-83, *83*
Calorie(s), burning off of, exercise guideline for, 73
  counting of, methods of, 65
  definition of, 42
  eating 1000 less per day, 63-64, 70
  functions of, 42
  insufficient, use of stored energy in, 42
  for maintenance of present weight, 63
  and nutrients, in refined and processed foods, 39
  for reducing of present weight, 63-64
  times 300, to reach training zone, 73
  for weekly weight loss, calculation of, 64
  working off of, to use fat, 70
Cancer, incidence of, 6
  lung, smoking as cause of, 22
Cannon, Walter B., and "fight or flight" response, 29
Carbohydrates, complex, in Well-Fit diet, 45
  composition of, 43
  daily intake of, in Well-Fit diet, 44
  uses of, in body, 43
Carpenter, Karen, 49
Chance, and medical problems, 104
Chest hugs, for stretching back, 80, *81*
Cigarette smoke/smoking. *See* Smoke; Smoking
Cigarettes, ads for, 24
Coffee, consumption of, annual, 26
Common sense, in nutrition, 41

Complacency, belief in myths leading to, 2, 3
Condition, 12-17
Control, sense of, and stress, 30, 33
Cooper, Kenneth, aerobics books by, 17
Cooper 12-Minute Test, 17
Coping, successful, 29
  with anxiety, 29
Cough, chronic, in smoking, 22
Cue avoidance, in behavior modification, 66
Curls, in strength training, *79*

Death, causes of, accepted by Americans, 6
  early, due to self-abuse, 6-8
  premature, cost of, 5
Denial, and mortality, 3
  use of, confidence in medicine and, 104
Dental cavities, cost of, 94
  development of, 95
  in U.S., 94
Dependency, in health care, 103-104
Diabetes, in obesity, 47
Diarrhea, in high carbohydrate diet, 98
Dairy, food, 66
Dickens, Charles, 8
Diet(s), American, 37
  and exercise, for weight loss, 69
  fad, 97-99
  health problems associated with, 18
  high carbohydrate, 98
  low carbohydrate, 98
  weight loss through, gaining back of, 69
  Well-Fit, 44-45
Diet aids, 99-100

Diet pills, 26-27, 99
Doctor(s), helping body to repair itself, 2
　and pills, 2
Drinking, in auto accidents, 6
　problems caused by, cost of, 5
　See also Alcohol, consumption of
Drugs, over-the-counter, 27
　prescription, 27
　recreational, 27
Dunn, Halbert, *High Level Wellness* by, 9

Earphone radios and cassette players, stress associated with, 30-31
Eating, as enjoyable, 36
　before bedtime, 62
　good, resource reading for, 45
　　Well-Fit Tips for, 45
　　　habits, good, in fitness program, 59
　　　industrialization and affluence influencing, 37
　　　modification of, 66-67
　　　poor, and results of, 40
　love of, history of, 36
　in moderation, 37
　reasons for, 66
　and unique tastes, development of, 36
Eating Log, use of, 66
Eating room, in behavior modification, 66
Emphysema, 7-8
　in smoking, 22
Employees, health of, as influence on business, 5-6
Exchange lists, resource reading on, 67
　in weight loss program, 65-66
Exercise(s), 52-54
　aerobic. *See* Aerobic exercise

　allowance for recovery from, 89
　as fun, 54
　avoidance of, 8
　bras for, 93
　correct approach to, 55
　couple of minutes per day, 101
　curls, *79*
　definitions of, 52
　diet and, for weight loss, 69
　during pregnancy, 92
　in fitness triad, 58, 59
　flyes, *78*
　functions of, 52-53
　heart rate, method of taking of, 57
　　training zone for, 55-56
　hyperextension, for back, *77, 78, 78*
　leg lowers, *76,* 77, *77*
　"is living," 52
　for lowering of weight set point, 64
　and menstruation, 92-93
　presses, *79*
　rational, in moderation, 83
　　resource reading for, 84
　　Well-Fit Way, 58, 59, 69-84
　regular, changes in body in, 52-53
　routine, to prevent over-use injury, 89
　safety of, 19
　situps, 75-77, *75, 76*
　for strength training of lower body, 74, *74, 75*
　and stress, 54
　for time-outs, 33
　triceps pushup, *80*
　twists, 78-79
　in weight loss program, 54
　Well-Fit, 55-57
　for women, misconceptions concerning, 93

Exercise program(s), persons at risk in, classification of, 19
  reading resources for, 20
  risk factors and, 18-19
  12-week, 72-73
Exercise study, incorrectly reported, 101

Fad diets, 97-99
Fads, 97-102
  resource reading on, 102
Failures, don't be afraid of, 11
Family, support of, weight loss program, 86-87
Fasts, protein sparing, 98-99
Fat(s), animal, 38
  in blood, as risk factor, 18-19
  body. *See* Body fat
  consumption, excess, and cancer, 40
    heart disease in, 40
    obesity in, 40
  daily intake of, in Well-Fit diet, 44, 45
  functions of, 43
  loss, from one area, products advertised for, 100
    study of, 100-101
  monosaturated, 38
  polyunsaturated, 38
  in red meat, 37-38
  saturated, 38
    problems associated with, 38
  sources of, in diet, 38
  stored, stimulation of body to use, 70
Fat body mass, 47
Fat cripple, 8
Fat percentage, definition of, 49
  determination of, 50-51
  in ideal range, maintenance of, 49-50

normal, 49
pathologic, 50
Fatty acid, essential, 43
Feedback, positive, in fitness program, 59-60
Feminine fitness, 92-93
Fetal alcohol syndrome, 25
Fiber, 39
"Fight or flight" response, 29
Fitness, assessment of, 16-17
  feminine, 92-93
  quickie, 101
Fitness program, change in, injury in, 89
  outside assistance in, 85-87
Fitness triad, 58-59
  finding time for, 60
  positive feedback in, 59-60
  resource reading for, 60
  rest in, 58, 59
  stress management in, 59
  weight regulation in, 58, 59
Flack, Roberta, 3
Flexibility training, stretching in, 80-83
Fluids, drinking of, 44
Flyes, in strength training, 78
Fonda, Jane, 10
Food(s), of American Indians, 37
  bad, 36-40
  creative, discovery of, 36
  flavoring of, development of, 37
  Industrial Revolution and, 37
  proteins in, 43
  refined, as harmful to teeth, 94
    and processed, 39-40
  supply, control over, development of, 36
  tastes, unique, development of, 36
  Well-Fit, 41-45
Food diary, 66
Food scale, in calorie counting, 65

Forks, use of, historical, 37
Four Free's in life, 2
Fractures, definition of, 91
   management in, 91
Friedman, Meyer, and Ray H. Rosenman, *Type A Behavior And Your Heart* by, 30, 32
Fructose, 38

Glucose, 38
Goals, realistic, setting of, 10
Group support, in behavior modification, 67
   for fitness training, 86
Gum disease, 95

HCG, as diet aid, 99–100
Health, comprehensive appraisal of, tests in, 17
   employee, as influence on business, 5–6
   fixing of, instantly, belief of, 2
   good, as expected, 9
      myths interfering with, 3–4
   improvement of, scope of benefits of, 11
   influence over, 1
   obsession with, as unhealthy, 11
Health care, cost of, 5
   dependency in, 103–104
   perfection in, belief in, 104
   self-responsibility for, 104
Health hazard appraisal, 12–14
   as advance in preventive medicine, 12
   risk factors examined in, 12–13
   Well-Fit lifestyle appraisal in, 13–14
Health problems, body fat and, 47–49
   caffeine and, 26
   related to eating habits, 40
   related to smoking, cost of, 22
Health spa(s), checking of, 86
   convenience of, need for, 85–86
   cost of, 85
   personnel, training of, checking of, 86
Heart, abnormalities of, as risk factor, 19, 88
   changes in, in long-term exercise, 53
   variation in, injury in, 88
Heart attack(s), incidence of, 6
   in young people, 7
Heart beat, resting, in long-term exercise, 53
Heart cripple, 8
Heart disease, in excess fat intake, 40
   incidence of, 6
   and obesity, 47
   risk factors for, 18–19
   and smoking, 22
Heart rate(s), exercising, highest, calculation of, 57
   lowest, calculation of, 57
   taking of, method of, 57
   maximum, calculation of, 55
   during exercise, 56
   resting, checking of, 15
   in long-term exercise, 53
   low, 57
   normal, 57
   training zone, calculation of, 56
Heart rate exercise training zone, 55–56
Height, measurement of, 14
High carbohydrate diets, 98
Home-Rahe Life Stress Scale, 30
Huang Ti, 9
Human chorionic gonadotropin, as diet aid, 99–100
Hyperextension, for strong back, 77, 78, *78*

INDEX

Hypertension. *See* Blood pressure, high

Ideal Body Weight (IBW), 50-51
  maintenance of, 64-65
Illness, cost of, 5
Improvement program, resource reading for, 60
  Well-Fit, 58-60
    finding time for, 60
    fitness triad in, 58-59
    positive feedback in, 59-60
    progress in, recording of, 59-60
Indians, American, food of, 37
Industrial Revolution, and food, 37
Infertility, smoking and, 22
INHTM syndrome, 3
Injury(ies), 88-91
  change in program causing, 89
  fractures as, 91
  in over-training, 89-90
  over-use, 89
  pain of, self-help in, 91
  resource reading on, 91
  strains and sprains as, 90
  in variation in anatomy, 88
Insulin, cellular sensitivity to, in obesity, 47
Italians, development of eating habits by, 37

Jogging, as aerobic exercise, 71

Ketosis, in low carbohydrate diets, 98
Knee hugs, for stretching back, 80, *81*
Knee problems, checking for, in exercise problem, 88
  strength training in, 74-75

Kobe beef, 37-38
Korbut, Olga, 50

Lean body mass, definition of, 46-47
Leg extension machine, *74, 75*
Leg extensions, finishing position for, *75*
  starting position for, 74
Leg lowers, in strength training, *76,* 77, *77*
Legs, lower, stretching of, 81-83, *83*
  upper backs of, stretching of, 80-81, *82*
Lieberman, E. James, on anxiety, 29, 32
Life, as free, 2
  as "package deal," 3
  Four Free's in, 2
Life expectancy, definition of, 10
  of men, 10
  and quality of, killing of, 5
  shortening of, through self-abuse, 10
  wellness and, 10
  of women, 10
Life span, definition of, 10
Lifestyle, bad, health problems associated with, 10
  family as influence on, 87
Linoleic acid, 43
Lipid Profile, 19
Log book, Eating, use of, 66
  of stress situations, 32
  Well-Fit, recording of daily calorie intake in, 65
Long Slow Distance (LSD) training, 56
Low back pain. *See* Back, low, pain in
Low carbohydrate diets, 98
"LSD," 56

Lung(s), cancer, smoking as cause of, 22
  compliancy of, in long-term exercise, 53
Lung cripple, breathing of, 6–7

Maximum heart rate, calculation of, 55
Mayer, Jean, on fad diets, 97
Meal(s), beginning and end, in behavior modification, 66
  long, in behavior modification, 67
Meat(s), protein from, 37–38
  red, and affluence, 37
  fat in, 37–38
  good qualities of, 38
Medical clearance, for exercise program, 19
Medical problems, chance and, 104
Medications. *See* Drugs
Medicine, modern, myths and, 3
  prospective, 9
Meditation, advantages of, 33–34
  during time-outs, 33
  easy method of, 34
  forms of, 34
  unifying influence following, 34
Menstruation, exercise and, 92–93
Methylxanthines. *See* Caffeine
Mind, in response to stress, 29
Minerals, 44
  "getting enough," 44
  uses of, in body, 43–44
Moderation, in good nutrition, 42
  in rational exercise, 83
Mortality, denial and, 3
Muscle(s), needing stretching, 80
  strain, 90
Myth(s), "can't-undertand," 1
  instant, every-problem-correction, 2
  interfering with good health, 3–4

modern medicine and, 3
mysterious, 1–4
"no-control-of-health," 1
"perfection is possible," 2–3

Neighborhood resources, 85–87
Nicotine addiction, 21, 23
Nutrients, 42–44
  and calories, in refined and processed foods, 39
  needed by body, 42
Nutrition, good, common sense in, 41
  moderation in, 42
  principles of, 41–42
  resource reading for, 45
  variety in, 41–42
  Well-Fit Tips for, 45

Obesity, combating of, 48
  contributing to heart disease, 47
  definition of, 16
  degenerative arthritis in, 48
  diabetes in, 47
  in excess fat intake, 40
  and high blood pressure, 6, 47
  incidence of, 46, 63
  low back pain in, 6
  management in, 8
1000-less-Calories-a-day technique, for weight loss, 64
Organizations, fitness programs of, 86
Over-the-counter drugs, 27
Over-training, over-use injury in, 89
  prevention of, monitoring in, 89–90
  symptoms of, 89
Over-use injury, 89

Pain, as signal of something wrong, 2–3

INDEX

feeling of own, 1
injury, self-help in, 91
low back, cost of, 5
obesity in, 6
Pelletier, Kenneth R., and meditation, 34
Periodontal disease, 95
Personality types, A and B, and stress, 30
Phenylpropanolamine, in diet pills, 99
  problems caused by, 27
  products containing, 26-27
Pickwickian syndrome, 8
Pill(s), diet, 26-27, 99
  "for every ill" myth, 2
Placebo, definition of, 100
Plaque, daily removal of, 95
  in dental cavities, 95
Polycyclic aromatic hydrocarbons (PAHs), as "ultimate carcinogens," 22
  in cigarette smoke, 22
  sources of, 22
Pregnancy, exercise during, 92
  smoking during, 22
Prescription drugs, 27
Presses, in strength training, 79
Problems, fixing, instantly, belief of, 2
Prospective medicine, 9
Protein(s), biological values of, in different foods, 43
  composition of, 43
  daily intake of, in Well-Fit diet, 44, 45
  essential, and daily requirements, 43
  functions of, 43
  from meat, 37-38
Protein sparing fasts, 98-99
Pulse, taking of, 15, *15*

Quickie fitness, 101

Recreational drugs, 27
Reducing Calories/day, calculation of, 63-64
Relaxation, smoking for, 23
Relaxation Response, of Herbert Benson, 34
  in reasonable rest, 62
Rest, in fitness triad, 58, 59, 61-62
Resting heart rate(s), checking of, 15
  in long-term exercise, 53
  low, 57
  normal, 57
Risk factors, and exercise program, 18-19
Rivers, Joan, on exercise, 8, 54
Rogers, Kenny, 12
Rosenman, Ray H., and Meyer Friedman, *Type A Behavior And Your Heart* by, 30, 32

Salt, as everywhere, 39
  too much, hazards of, 39
Self-abuse, shortening of life expectancy through, 10
Self-help, in injury pain, 91
Situps, in strength training, 75-77, *75*, *76*
Skin-fold measurements, in determination of fat percentage, 50
Skin problems, in sun exposure, 96
Sleep, development of routine for, 61
  eating before, 62
  relaxation before, 62
Smoke, cigarette, carcinogens in, 22
Smoking, 21-24
  addiction to nicotine in, 21, 23
  ads for, 24
  as "keeping hands busy" habit, 23
  as physical addiction, 21

as psychological habit, 21
as risk factor, 18
during pregnancy, 22
health problems related to, cost of, 22
and heart disease, 22
immediate effects of, 21–22
incidence of, 22
and infertility, 22
long-term effects of, 22
quitting of, 8
  belief in self for, 23
  exercise and, 54
  group help for, 23, 24
  on own, suggestions for, 23
reasons for, 23
stopping. *See* Smoking, quitting of
Snacking, prevention of, in behavior modification, 66, 67
Spas, health. *See* Health spa(s)
Spot reducing products, 100–101
Sprain(s), definition of, 90
  sites of, 90
  treatment of, 90
Sputum production, in smoking, 22
Starch blockers, 100
Starvation, use of stored energy in, 42
Stimulant(s), caffeine as, 26
  nicotine as, 23
Strain(s), definition of, 90
  in response of mind to stress, 29
  sites of, 90
  treatment of, 90
Strength training, and aerobic exercise, 73
  areas of focus in, 74
  gradual working up to, 73
  of lower body, 74
    in knee problems, 74–75
  progressive increase in resistance in, 73

of trunk, 75–79, *75, 76, 77, 78*
of upper body, *78,* 79, *79,* 80
Stress, 28–31
appraisal of, and reaction to, 30
as necessary part of life, 32
coping with, 28–29
  in body, 29
definition of, 28
exercise in management of, 54
good and bad things causing, 30–31
handling of, improvement in methods of, 30
helpful, 32–35
log book of situations causing, 32
long-term, as harmful, 29–30
  sickness following, 30
management of, in fitness program, 59, 61, 62
psychological, 29
reaction to, appraisal of, as influence on, 30
resource reading on, 31
and sense of control, 30, 33
Well-Fit, 32–35
  resource reading on, 35
Stress test(s), 16–17
for exercise program, 19
Stretching, in flexibility training, 80–83
Stretching activities, in exercise program, 70–71, 73
Stroke, incidence of, 6
Sugar, as everywhere, 38, 39
composition of, 38
daily consumption of, 39
Sun, exposure of skin to, diseases associated with, 96
skin problems associated with, 96
Swimming, as aerobic exercise, 71
Synergism, definition of, 69

INDEX

3/10 Principle, explanation of, 69
Time management, in coping with stress, 33
Time-outs, daily, activities during, 33
  need for, 33
  exercise during, 33
Tobacco industry, ads of, 24
Tooth(Teeth), decay, cost of, 94
  development of, 95
  in U.S., 94
  good, care necessary for, 94, 95
Trace elements, 44
  uses of, in body, 43-44
Training, Long Slow Distance (LSD), 56
  strength. *See* Strength training
Training zone, heart rate exercise, 55-56
  heart rate in, calculation of, 56
  300 calorie times, to reach, 73
Treadmill, stress test, for exercise program, 19
Triceps pushups, in strength training, *80*
Trunk, strength training for, 75-79, *75, 76, 77, 78*
Twists, to exercise trunk, 78-79
Type A Behavior And Your Heart, by Friedman and Rosenman, 30, 32

Under-water weight, in determination of fat percentage, 50

Variety, in nutrition, 41-42
Vitamin(s), 44
  "getting enough," 44
  megadoses of, 102
  natural and synthetic, 102
  necessary daily amount of, 101
  supplementation, 102
  uses of, in body, 43-44

Waist, circumference, measurement of, 14
Walking, as aerobic exercise, 71
Water, balance, maintenance of, 44
  loss, in low carbohydrate diets, 98
  weight loss from losing, 64
Weight, assessment of, 14
  Ideal Body (IBW), 50-51
  maintenance of, 64-65
  gain, following loss through diet, 69
  loss, diet and exercise for, 69
  exercise program for, 54
  in fad diets, 97
  from losing water, 64
  lowering of weight set point for, 64
  per week, calories for, calculation of, 64
  spot reducing products for, 100-101
  through diet, gaining back of, 69
  present, maintenance of, calories for, 63
  reducing of, calories for, 63-64
  regulated, Well-Fit point, 67
  in Well-Fit Way, 63-68
  regulation of, in fitness triad, 58, 59
  set point, lowering of, 64
  Well-Fit, 49-51
Weight loss centers, 86
Well-Fit diet, 44-45
Well-Fit exercise, 55-57
Well-Fit food, 41-45
Well-Fit life, acceptance of failures in, 11
  basis of, 105
  good teeth as necessary for, 94-95
  moderation in health focus of, 11
  new viewpoint for, 11

and quality of life, 103
realistic goals for, 10
time-outs in, 33
Well-Fit Lifestyle Appraisal, 13
scoring of, 13-14
Well-Fit log book, recording of daily calorie intake in, 65
Well-Fit program, 58-60
Well-Fit Tips, for alcohol and drug use, 27
for assessment of neighborhood resources, 87
for attaining ideal body weight, 51
for care of body parts, 94-96
concerning body fat, 48
for control of health, 4
on eating, 40
on exercise, 54
on fads, 102
on feminine fitness, 93
for good eating, 45
for good exercise, 57
for good life, 104
on health appraisal, 17
for health maintenance, 8
for improvement program, 60
for prevention of injury, 91
prior to exercise, 20
for rational exercise, 84
for reasonable rest, 62
for stopping smoking, 24
stress and, 31
and stress as necessary part of life, 34
for weight regulation, 67
for wellness, 11
Well-Fit Way, exercise in, 58, 59, 69-84
12-week program of, 72-73
reasonable rest in, 58, 59, 61-62
regulated weight in, 63-68
Well-Fit weight, 49-51
Wellness, 9-11
approach to life, 9
as health with few limitations, 9
benefits of, 9-10
and life expectancy, 10
Wishful thinking, and correction of problems, 2

YMCA and YWCA, spas in, 86